Crip Screens

Crip Screens

Countering Psychiatric Media Technologies

OLIVIA BANNER

Duke University Press   *Durham and London*   2025

© 2025 DUKE UNIVERSITY PRESS. All rights reserved
Project Editor: Bird Williams
Designed by Courtney Leigh Richardson
Typeset in Warnock Pro by Copperline Book Services

Library of Congress Cataloging-in-Publication Data
Names: Banner, Olivia author
Title: Crip screens : counter psychiatry / Olivia Banner.
Description: Durham : Duke University Press, 2025. |
Includes bibliographical references and index.
Identifiers: LCCN 2025009900 (print)
LCCN 2025009901 (ebook)
ISBN 9781478032564 paperback
ISBN 9781478029205 hardcover
ISBN 9781478061397 ebook
Subjects: LCSH: Mental health services—Technological
innovations | Mental health services—Information
technology | Sociology of disability | Internet in
psychotherapy | Internet in medicine | Mental
illness—Treatment | Psychotherapy—echnological
innovations
Classification: LCC RC480.5 .B3225 2025 (print)
LCC RC480.5 (ebook)
DDC 362.20285—dc23/eng/20250804
LC record available at https://lccn.loc.gov/2025009900
LC ebook record available at https://lccn.loc.gov/2025009901

Cover art: Courtesy Adobe Stock/klikk and Allusioni.

To the spillover and
to the streets

Contents

INTRODUCTION

The Spillover and Psychiatric Ways of Screening

It was Ella, Ella,
queen Ella had come
and words spilled out
... whose voice lingers on
that stage gone mad with
perdido perdido
i lost my heart in toledooooooooo
—SONIA SANCHEZ, "A Poem for Ella Fitzgerald"

In 2022, California offered two illuminating examples of what this book names psychiatric ways of screening. The California legislature signed into law the Community Assistance, Recovery, and Empowerment (CARE) Act, which allows for the forced incarceration and medication of so-called mentally ill people who match a list of criteria, one of which is certain diagnoses outlined in the *Diagnostic and Statistical Manual of Mental Disorders* (DSM), psychiatry's bible of diagnostic screening that is now in its fifth revised version. Although the DSM is an old psychiatric instrument, it is an endlessly updatable instrument, readied for revision every decade, and, in the case of the CARE Act, it is an instrument of incarceration. Also in 2022, researchers in the University of California Los Angeles (UCLA) Department of Psychiatry framed their study that gave undergraduate enrollees iPhones and AppleWatches to record biodata, including about their sleep, as "moderniz[ing] mental health" and "bring[ing] mental health into the 21st century."[1] Cops in the streets, tech bros in the sheets—psychiatric ways of screening come in many disguises and serve multiple masters. In each new revision, in each new technological form, they serve to occlude the crisis of care produced from racial capitalism and its henchmen, the medical-industrial complex and the technology industries' extraction of value from human sociality.

This book will argue that such psychiatric ways of screening are psychiatry's response to widespread social and cultural challenges to its authority. Psychiatry responded to 2020's worldwide protests against racial injustice and policing with claims that technological innovation could right its historical enmeshment with these systems: psychiatric ways of screening would substitute for the discipline's ongoing failures to fulfill its mission to understand and treat "mental illness." This book's archive demonstrates that this has historically been the response of psychiatry, as well as its related disciplines, professions, and institutions, what is called here the psy-ences. Moments of challenges to psychiatry's authority and disciplinary power over the populations it racially pathologizes have been met with lofty claims that technology can heal the psy-ences' decay and with accompanying efforts to technologize the disciplines and their clinical practice. Existing alongside these efforts, the people that they have racially pathologized have engaged in what I call counter-psychiatric practices of media and technology activism. The archive of minor media and activism that this book explores illuminates a counter psychiatry that diverges from a popular culture–dominant imaginary that narrates psychiatry's challengers as "anti" and as white-led. This archive demonstrates a crip genealogy of a counter psychiatry articulated within the sphere of cultural production.

The crip genealogy this book illuminates did not structure itself as oppositional to psychiatry, as did the antipsychiatry movement and the countercultural movements that favored "alternative therapies." The crip genealogy unearthed here often did not even explicitly engage with any instances of psychiatric, psychologistic, or professional therapeutic clinical practice, or even with their discourses. This crip genealogy played out within the sphere of media and technology, as those subject to the state's and psychiatry's pathologizing visions and debilitating practices sought to envision care, and deliver it, otherwise. The moments of cultural production this book ushers to the fore used the tools at hand to explore and construct visions of care for people in distress that did not depend on or traffic with psy discourses and their institutional manifestations. They cannot, therefore, be called "antipsychiatry"— their practice eschewed capture within the terms the psy-ences laid out for those experiencing mental distress. This book calls them, instead, crip screens, whose logic was to counter psychiatry and its ways of screening.

Psychiatric ways of screening include the media screens on which representational narratives appear: from the mental hygiene films shown in midcentury high schools to the smartphone on which you watch cognitive behavioral therapy (CBT) videos. They also include the informatic schemas, data regimes, and computational logics that distinguish among and classify symptoms, diagnoses, populations, and risk. These include, for example, the big data episteme that allows a third-party company to use the fact that you accessed a CBT video to change your credit score based on your presumed "mental health." To summarize, in this book, *psychiatric ways of screening* are the entangled media, technologies, and psy-ences that prop up continued discursive and financial investment in those disciplines and that secure their power to enforce biopolitics, via their authority to construct categories and hierarchies of difference. They exist in relation to the phantasms conjured by psychiatry, those presumed risks and dysfunctions of unruly people, which psychiatry exists to contain.

Although this book's chapters home in on the 1960s and 1970s, I introduce its central concepts, themes, and practices by reading through an example from the 1930s. While an outlier to the main historical era of the chapters' archive, this example demonstrates the longer arc of the history of psychiatric ways of screening. To be sure, that arc extends much farther back in historical time, and so I could have reached for others; but due to its main character's relevance to later chapters and its technological innovation's centrality to psyentific research today, it is not as random as it might appear. It describes the origin of network science, a branch of theory that underpins and fuels social-networking sites, national security regimes that use metadata about digital communications to target humans for murder by drone or for incarceration, and various avenues of research in psychiatry and neuroscience. Many publications about network science note that Jacob Moreno innovated the network graph in the early twentieth century and move on to their next point. These accounts elide the setting for Moreno's research: a segregated girls' prison, the New York State Hudson Training School for Girls. Restoring to this origin story its full context reveals that psychiatric ways of screening cohere through informatic and visual logics that enact racialized and antiqueer violence, defining as ungovernable that which their epistemes seek to govern.[2]

As feminist historians have shown, under wayward girls' laws, these Progressive Era prisons incarcerated both Black and queered working-class girls and enforced reformers' ideologies about the impropriety of working-class family life, enacting an antiqueer, anti-Black platform.[3] Moreno, already attracting notoriety for his therapeutic technique known as "psychodramatic theater" and with one other prison research study (at Sing Sing Prison) under his belt, was invited by Hudson's superintendent, Fannie French Morse, to conduct research at Hudson, with the ostensible aim of improving Hudson's program of rehabilitation. This is how Morse described the prison's rehabilitative aims: "The spill-over, or seeking for the exploitation of adventure and thrill, has brought the average delinquent girl to the institution. Her rehabilitation must come, not through the elimination of these forces, but a substitute. It must come from the ramming out of the old with a new and bigger and more thrilling, a more vivid and more unique interest than the old.... To this adventurous girl who, seeking for adventure many times has brought her a delinquent to the institution, there is nothing like the stunt or project."[4] As we shall see, this rehabilitation was as segregated as all other parts of the prison: white "average delinquent girls" were given a "more vivid and unique interest" in the form of working on the farm, or singing in a choir; Black girls imprisoned in Hudson had their "spill-over" "rammed out" through steam-laundry work, where the girls often sustained third-degree burns, or through solitary confinement in the basements of their segregated cottages, where they were often subjected to beatings by prison staff. It is no wonder that when Moreno arrived at Hudson, there was an "outbreak of runaways," as he put it, or, as we might put it, a refusal of forced rehabilitation with fugitivity.

Moreno's book *Who Shall Survive? A New Approach to the Problem of Human Interrelations* (1934) reported on his two years of research at the prison. *Who Shall Survive?* sets out its central goal as producing a science of the sociology of group relations, in order that "a true therapeutic procedure" could take "the whole of mankind" as its object and thus build "harmonious communities."[5] It had two goals, then: design a science of group relations, including of those who constituted Morse's spillover, and craft a therapeutic program that would improve each group's relations. Moreno's vision of groups and their capacities for harmonious social relations was eugenic, even as he appeared to eschew the more typical direct interventions into breeding; he described as primitive groups that did not allow for spontaneous creativity, and as modern (industrial capitalist) those that did. His eugenics took as its target developing the best groups, which he defined as those in which individuals were freed to express their spontaneous creativity and thus best contribute to productive labor.[6]

Moreno created "sociometric tests" to measure "attractions and repulsions" among the girls. While one chief aim of the tests was to stop fugitivity, his descriptions of these attractions and repulsions centered on ensuring heteronormative development in the white girls, which was, in his thinking, threatened by the potentially queer, if interracial, possibilities of these friendship currents. In other words, Moreno posed Black girls as queering heteronormative development. A central moment when Moreno establishes that his system is a true science arrives in a section of the book filled with visualizations, with the climactic one included as figure I.1, titled "Psychological Geography of a Community." Throughout this book I attempt to provide rich description in addition to alt-text, but this particular image stymies rich description. It looks like one of my doodles—like a child's scribble, or initial work in an art class about creating shadows. Perhaps it charts the movement of ships in the transatlantic slave trade. It contains fourteen circles connected by many lines. When there are more lines, the particular route between circles appears darker, stronger. Perhaps it is a diagram for threads: a cat's cradle, or a basket. But Moreno describes it as a psychological geography, a visibilizing map of invisible terrain, so for now we will go with that.[7] With this image, Moreno cements his claim: His science allows him to map, to visualize through abstractions, the emotional currents circulating through the different cottages in which the girls lived.

Moreno claimed that the science he had innovated allowed him to deduce which girls and which cottage groups spurred the most emotional attractors. When new prisoners arrived at Hudson, Moreno would administer his sociometric test, apply his particular abstracted logic of currents, and assign them to a cottage—recall that these were segregated—best suited for maintaining order within these emotional currents. This, he claimed, stopped the outbreak of runaways—his applied science achieved carceral success. That his science innovated a psychiatric way of screening—a technology that separated and made distinctions in order to mark out who was rehabilitatable—crystallizes in a section about the steam laundry. Claiming there had been "racial riots" in the steam laundry, he pinpointed Stella, a Black girl, as the key troublemaker there—apparently Stella's spillover was not yet "rammed out" of her. Moreno recommended that Stella be moved to a different work group, and, after she was relocated, Moreno claimed the "racial riots" that had

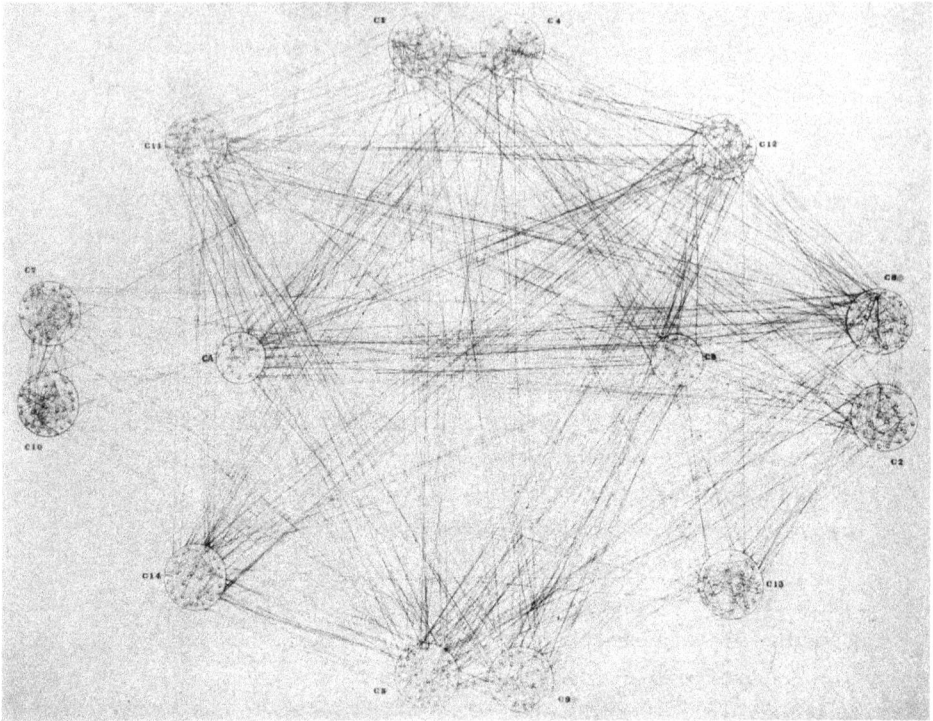

FIGURE I.1. "Psychological Geography of a Community" by Jacob Moreno, from *Who Shall Survive?* (1934).

occurred settled down. He evidenced this claim through two visualizations, seen in figure I.2. The image on the left visualizes attractions and repulsions within the steam laundry during Stella's spillover. The image on the right visualizes these after Stella was removed. (Actually, the evocative terms Moreno uses are "before re-construction" and "after re-construction.") The differences in the visualizations are fairly unremarkable, except for the fact that the right image ("post re-construction") features more "red" lines, which signify attractions. Obviously, this is all silly—any industrial boss would cast off the factory floor an organizer or someone challenging oppressive labor conditions. If Stella appeared to be organizing workers against each other or against the forewoman, or if Stella raised her voice against their dangerous working conditions, no factory owner or forewoman needed science to inform their next action. Moreno's achievement with these visualizations was to morph common knowledge into a system of informatics that could be used, revised, and

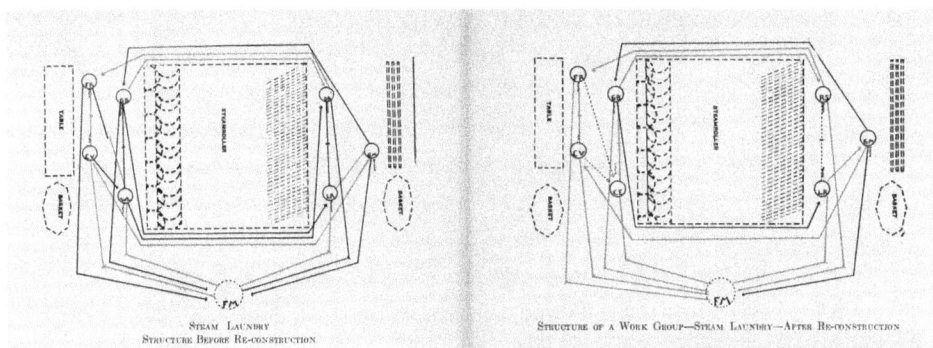

FIGURE I.2. Visualizations of the "psychogeography" of the steam laundry: on the left, with Stella; on the right, without Stella. From Jacob Moreno, *Who Shall Survive?* (1934).

operationalized to govern unruliness and enhance anti-Black and ableist discourses of economic productivity.

Instituted in a segregated prison and in a research study where Black girls' presumed queerness threatened the presumed heterosexuality of white girls, these graphs abstracted the queered color line into a racialized data regime.[8] The innovation of the network graph arose specifically to contain fugitive currents—girls who fled a prison; Black-led resistance to dangerous work conditions—and to ensure white heteronormativity.

Moreno also produced a silent film of his applied program of therapy, which he presented at various prestigious universities to promote his work. The film showed Moreno conducting therapy with only the white girls at the prison: it representationally produced the proper subject for rehabilitation as the white girl. These two psychiatric ways of screening, the network graph and the promotional film, erased Black girls from the scene of rehabilitation—the media and technologies ungendered Black girls, removing them from the scene of rehabilitation.[9] The network graph performed the work of eugenic biopolitics, reproducing a hierarchy of racialized and queered pathologies, deployed to shore up categories of racialized difference. It abstracted into a visualization of nodes and edges in use, today, for classifying into gendered and racialized types, entrenching inequalities, and reproducing racialized violence. It made the law informatic; it made informatics the American grammar book.

Even though banished from the phantasm of spontaneous creativity in Moreno's imaginings, those girls continued to pursue their own "stunts and projects," flexing their creativity to escape the prison's confines, even as Moreno pronounced his prison therapeutic program successful.[10] Among them was Ella Fitzgerald, sentenced for the crime of being "ungovernable" and incarcerated while Moreno was at Hudson. Fitzgerald escaped the prison and returned to Harlem. Such were "the stunts" and "the projects" that adventurous, thrill-seeking girls pursued: lives of freedom, liberated from the racialized violence of Progressive-era interventions; such was their spillover. I steal the term *spillover* from Morse, not so much as an act of recovery but for how aptly it indicates the threat that girls, especially Black girls, were constructed to pose to structures of difference and the ontological (and material) walls erected to shore up their boundaries.

Throughout this book I mobilize *spillover* to evoke the excess that always already escapes psy-entific logic, and/yet that the psy-ences require to legitimate their projects. In the instance of Hudson, the spillover tethers itself to Black girls and their supposed threat to normative white (hetero)reproductivity. Although many of the psychiatric ways of screening elaborated in this book do indeed circle around Black girls, within the cultural works I analyze, as the social movements of the 1960s grew more complicated and interdependent, sometimes the spillover adumbrates a broader scope of populations designated as needing governing. Often psychiatry viewed those critical of psychiatry as the spillover—constituting a threat to the disciplinary enterprise itself. As Morse used the term specifically in relation to young women, I admit that for my project Morse's term is imperfect. Yet Morse's own imprecision defining it—her repetitions, her euphemisms, her evasions—also signals how vast she conceived of the slippery force she sought to contain, that indefinability of young girls riffing on, jangling among, and refusing regulatory regimes that sought to capture them.

In the long 1960s, psychiatric ways of screening developed out of the need to construct a spillover to justify psychiatry's ongoing expansions. These psychiatric ways of screening have been informed by psychiatry's specific disciplinary quandary: its continued tenuous grasp on authority and knowledge. Owen Whooley argues that the discipline's ignorance about what constitutes "mental illness"—an ignorance that throws its status as science into doubt— produces cycles of crisis and reinvention. This book argues that media and technological invention are core to the reinvention phase. To underline this, I will illustrate another psychiatric way of screening that arose during the heightened period of social crises on which this book centers, the 1960s and 1970s. It is psychologist Paul Ekman's Facial Action Coding System (FACS), a typology of facial expressions claimed to be universal and machine-readable. Its origin story, as told by Ekman, critics of FACS, and historians of science and technology, is that it emerged from its era's anthropological structuralism combined with a US Department of Defense (DOD) goal to fund lie-detection technologies.[11] These stories elide what some might consider to be the main reason for the DOD's interest—the explosion of third world liberation struggles worldwide and the US state's ongoing surveillance of those designated dangerous to law and order. These origin stories also overlook that Ekman's initial research occurred at a mental institution—the perfect carceral laboratory by which to make the social technological.

Ekman's earliest research centered on creating a technology that would enable researchers to search for and retrieve information across vast archives of film and videotape. The system he developed, Visual Information Display and Retrieval (VID-R), linked videotape recorders and monitors to a teletype machine and a computer. An operator would watch the visual recordings and code the expressions made by the people recorded. These people were psychiatric patients held in wards at Langley Porter Neuropsychiatric Institute, in San Francisco, California. Ekman's earliest publications about VID-R do not name exactly which videotapes he used—in other words, it's unclear whether he took existing videotapes from other research going on in Langley Porter, including the experiment I discuss in chapter 1, or he recorded new videotapes of patients. In his autobiography, he indicates that he filmed interviews of depressed patients at Langley upon their admission and release, suggesting those might be the recordings.[12] Whether he used videotape he had recorded or reused other recordings is, perhaps, inconsequential to the bigger takeaway: At Langley, videotaping patients was standard practice, and it was in a mental ward that Ekman joined computational technologies to visualizing technologies, toward the ultimate goal of developing a technology that could distinguish among affective comportments and detect pathologies: a psychiatric way of screening.[13] In his autobiography, Ekman relates that psychiatric residents at Langley asked Ekman, then focused on a typology of facial expressions from photographs and film from Margaret Mead's New Guinea site, if he could identify whether a patient, admitted for a suicide attempt and requesting a weekend pass, was lying about improved mental status. It was this question, with its core interest in distinguishing among deceit and psychiatric status, that inspired his idea of a high-speed video system with computational logic. Funded through the DOD, Ekman and an engineer spent eighteen months at Langley Porter to produce VID-R.[14]

Should we care about Ekman's earliest media-technological innovations at a psychiatric ward, which historians have largely ignored? I argue that we should. While Ekman's prior research lab was the colony, here, Ekman moved his lab to the psychiatric ward. Those deemed outside the human (in the colony, non-Westerners; in the psychiatric ward, spillovers of the irrational and the illogical) served as proving grounds for a psychiatric way of screening that could *make distinctions*—in the case of lie-detecting technologies, between truth and lies, friends and enemies of the state; in the case of psychiatric technologies, between "mental illness" and "mental health," the abnormal and the normal—and become computable. For the next two decades of Ekman's career, working with the IT professions and the CIA, Ekman made his pathologizing system fully computational.

That his psychiatric way of screening imposes its system of governance as a racial pathologizing project is evident in the most banal of today's technologies, from its use by first-world airport security screeners to screen out supposed terrorist threats to third-party employment firms that promise to use it to screen for "employable" applicants. In 2019, HireVue, a "hire tech" company, announced a new feature of its software, which enables job applicants to use a computer or other device with video-recording features to record their answers to job application interview questions. This new feature was an "emotional assessment algorithm," which HireVue claimed could "read" people's facial expressions to decode their emotional states, which would presumably "predict" which applicants would succeed at the applied-for position. On social media, critics immediately pointed out the normative biases underpinning such assessments, in particular how they might interpret neurodivergent people as deceptive, pathological, or otherwise unworthy of being hired. They additionally decried that, because facial recognition technologies have been trained on racist datasets and cannot accurately map data points on the faces of people with darker skin, HireVue's algorithm would be biased toward light-skinned people as manifesting "readable"—in this case, employable—faces. Threatened with legal challenges, HireVue retracted the software.

Like the racializing technology of the network graph, such "emotional algorithm" software reinstates a socius where whiteness is capacitated.[15] Like the network graph now applied for police surveillance, this software arose from within a setting of carceral pathologization. This is what Cristina Mejia Visperas calls "science in captivity": research and technological innovation that seeks out so-called contained settings—the prison and the ward—under a justification that a controlled environment decreases the variables affecting the experiment and allows the scientist a clearer view of the workings of nature.[16] Yet the prison and the ward are social arrangements. Psychiatric ways of screening transmute social arrangements into technologies of control. They recuperate legitimacy for disciplines beset by constant epistemological and cultural crises. They claim for these disciplines the scienticity of technology while reproducing older and producing new operations of anti-Blackness and ableism.[17]

Crip Genealogies and Counter-Psychiatric Histories

There is an abundance of work on cultures of psychiatry and antipsychiatry from those trained in history, sociology, science and technology studies, and cultural studies. Increasingly too there are histories about the creation of automated and digital diagnoses.[18] Unlike those, this book approaches its topic through a feminist-of-color disability analytic that informs the crip genealogy it establishes. Drawing from woman-of-color feminists such as Audre Lorde, Gloria Anzaldúa, Sami Schalk, and Jina Kim, it develops a feminist-of-color disability analytic that "[attends] to the linkages between the ideologies of ability and the logics of gender and sexual regulation that undergird racialized resource deprivation . . . that is, how ableist violence operates alongside and through heteropatriarchy, capitalism, and white supremacy."[19] Along with policing and schools, Schalk and Kim name prisons as key "instruments of mass disablement [disproportionately targeting] black and brown populations."[20] *Crip Screens* centers the state apparatus and discourse of psychiatry within this analysis, arguing that its technologies have functioned as immaterial instrumentalizations of mass disablement. Morse's spillover placed in particular young Black girls at the center of structures of disablement; Moreno's network graph constituted an abstracted instrument of disablement predicated on the queered color line and the (white) heteroreproductivity necessary for social reproduction and surplus labor.

For a feminist-of-color disability analytic, activism against such instruments of mass disablement remains a key site of theorizing their dismantling. This book follows the spillover's "stunts," its avenues of flight, that were encoded in works of cultural production. These cultural works often explicitly countered psychiatric ways of screening and their racial pathologizing discourses; sometimes, echoing La Marr Jurelle Bruce's *How to Go Mad Without Losing Your Mind*, they strategically inhabited discourses of racial pathologization.[21] I explore moments when the human subjects of these data regimes both openly challenged and implicitly resisted them. This opens up a deeper genealogy of resistance to psychiatry's technology modernizing projects. This analytic reveals determined efforts by those regulated within classifying systems of gender, sexuality, ability, sanism, and race to challenge psychiatry's carcerality and violence, including the media technologies through which it has constantly reasserted its authority. It opens up a crip genealogy for counter-psychiatric histories.

A crip genealogical method means archival practice that reads against the grain, follows trails where they flash out from beneath the surface, and muddies some disciplinary tendencies. I opened this introduction with Moreno's inauguration contribution to the development of the informatic subject and will conclude it with Ella Fitzgerald's encoding of crip worldmaking in her early career for two reasons: first, to offer one model of how this book reads cultural production; second, due to the intransigent fact that, of all US states, the state of New York archived its prisons' records extensively, affording historical excavations for feminist, queer, and Black studies. New York City plays an outsized role in this book, a function of its history as an urban location in which so many US state policies were tested and realized, in which media and computational industries flourished, and in which activist cultures and subcultures thrived—including within archival institutions responsible for preserving cultural works. It is my hope that some of the archival discoveries this book makes will inspire others to continue seeking out crip genealogies beyond the confines of the archive of cultural texts assembled here, which do not extend beyond the late 1970s.

While this book may make modest contributions to the fields on which it draws—histories of psychiatry, media studies, film studies, and critical studies of data culture—those are incidental to its central contribution to crip genealogies and cultural studies. Still, it is worth noting the recent scholarship in the history of the psy-ences that revisit their ongoing crises, including Lucas Richert's *Break on Through*, Owen Whooley's *On the Heels of Ignorance*, and Michael Staub's *Madness Is Civilization*, on which this book draws. To differing degrees, these works hover around the disciplines' and professions' internal debates; I hope that this book enriches these discussions through its attention to the external pressures that shaped them. Film studies is also rich in scholarship about therapy, psychiatry, and psychology; I hope that this book opens up more discussions about insurgent, crip, and independent Black film practices.[22] Finally, this book converses with critical feminist, queer, and Black data studies work that has opened up counterhistories of computation, information, and technologies.

Crip Worldmaking Beyond Violent
Racialized Data Regimes

Today, disability communities engage in organizing and mutual aid efforts to imagine and establish worlds that value and support, and help crip flourishing, thereby "worldmaking" beyond our current regime of necropolitical ableism, racism, sexism, and colonialism.[23] As a model of the readings to come, I want to return, here, to Ella Fitzgerald. While Fitzgerald's life and music have been well documented in jazz histories, the earliest part of her career, just after she spilled out of the prison, is occluded within these histories. Here, I reconstruct this clouded history as one of crip worldmaking.

Fitzgerald's first point of postincarceration worldmaking began through a partnership with the crippled band leader and drummer Chick Webb. A self-taught drummer, Webb had tuberculosis of the spine, resulting in what an article in the music magazine *Down Beat* described as his "deformed, dwarfish, and delicate" appearance.[24] In *Drummin' Men*, a multivolume history of jazz drummers, Webb's entry—the book's first entry, due to his significance within jazz drumming—is studded with descriptions of his hunchback, whether they were taken from oral histories or quoted from music reviews published at the time.[25] Webb was a legend in jazz circles, innovating entirely new methods of drum play, and his allegiance to his struggling bandmates caused him to turn down higher-paying gigs with Duke Ellington, among others. When it became clear that a female vocalist would strengthen the band's appeal, contacts urged him to meet Fitzgerald, who, at the time, was living on the streets and busking on 125th Street. Descriptions of their initial meetings highlight Fitzgerald's unkempt, nonheteronormative appearance. She is called ugly, too big to fit the mold of seductive female vocalists, unwashed, and uncombed. No matter those descriptions, however, as all Webb needed was to hear her singing voice and she was hired. He got her housed. Quickly, the Chick Webb band, with Fitzgerald fronting, had commercial success. Fitzgerald was eighteen years old. Within four years, Webb's tuberculosis would overcome him, forcing him into multiple hospital stays and, eventually, death.

The partnership between these two Black musicians, one "unfit" and one "ungovernable," was a form of crip worldmaking. Fitzgerald had managed to escape twice from prisons (before Hudson, she had escaped another girls' prison). She was found and recognized by a drummer who surely knew that his physical status placed him always in danger of being forced into medically racist institutional settings, if not dependency on a state that would debilitate him through its racist modes of care. Together, for the four years preceding his death, they supported each other, living under the threat of incarceration.

Viewing their partnership as a survival of crip worldmaking, I now illustrate my method of theorizing through cultural works by turning to recover their musical productions that jazz historians have dismissed. Although Fitzgerald was an immensely popular performer and singer, jazz historians have not praised her and Webb's early output. Critical music studies historian Christi J. Wells explains that this occurred even in their own lifetime. Webb had come, for some music critics, to embody Black anticommercialism; when he added Fitzgerald to the band, and together they had commercially successful and supposedly "unserious" hits, critics viewed her as detracting from his anticommercial and artistic possibilities.[26] Wells also argues that even if succeeding generations of jazz historians laud Fitzgerald's vocal style, sophisticated syncopation, and general contributions to jazz, they have reproduced this disdain for her in representing her as a feminized distraction from the important masculine business of "real" art. Wells contextualizes this dismissal within the homosociality of jazz and the denigrated femininity of Fitzgerald's presence and contribution to the band (where a "voice" was seen as feminine and thus lesser than instruments, which were seen as masculine). Yet at least one of her early works, "A-Tisket A-Tasket," slyly, subtly, and spillingly signified on how incarceration had cripped her—how being a young Black girl in America immediately subjected her to racialized and gendered systems of violence. Although this book is not addressed to jazz historians, here I recover that most dismissed of her songs as a work with a serious subtext, one that commented on systems of oppression.

Fitzgerald composed "A-Tisket A-Tasket" for Webb during one of his many illnesses.[27] It is a song from one crip to another. A reinterpretation of a traditional child's play song, "A-Tisket A-Tasket" takes what is typically classified as "children's stuff"—not adult, not-yet-citizen, small, relegated to music's remainder bin—and flips it for serious themes. In crip theoretical terms, it re-values a devalued form and does so with a richly coded irony. The lyrics signify on the numbers game and the criminalization of Blackness occurring through police protection of non-Black runners, thus indicating Fitzgerald's own pathologized childhood, when she was arrested for numbers running and sent to her first prison. They also signify on "mama's baby, papa's maybe," the racialized American grammar by which biological familial ties were interrupted and not-yet-reproductive girls were ungendered, left to project their spontaneous routes out of their prisons.

A-Tisket A-Tasket
A brown and yellow basket
I sent a letter to my mommie
On the way I dropped it
I dropped it, I dropped it
Yes, on the way I dropped it
A little girlie picked it up
And put it in her pocket
She was truckin' on down the Avenue
Without a single thing to do
She was peck, peck, peckin' all around
When she spied it on the ground
She took it, she took it
My little yellow basket
And if she doesn't bring it back
I think that I will die . . .

While the song begins with "A brown and yellow basket," the remainder of the song's lyrics mention only yellow: Its brown descriptor drops out. I read the initial description of "brown and yellow" as referring to colorism, something Sonia Sanchez would draw out in "A Poem for Ella Fitzgerald," where Sanchez names "high-steppin' yellers" to allude to the colorism that characterized high and low culture at the time.[28] Once imprisoned in Moreno's contained laboratory for therapeutic research, colorism intensified. According to Moreno, at Hudson "darker girls" were favored over lighter-skinned girls, and when a light-skinned girl, Jane, insulted Stella's mother, a group of darker girls supported Stella during their subsequent disagreement. If we want to interpret the song as signifying on Fitzgerald's time at Hudson, perhaps its cheerful and playful mode gestures to her fugitive freedom, that she had broken free of a prison situation that pitted racialized girls against each other.

In the song, the basket is also connected to sending a letter to a mother. Here, historical contextualization reveals more of the song's signifying. Hyman Kassell was a widely known successful operator of numbers running in Harlem; he owned speakeasies during Prohibition, and, at the time of the song's composition, he operated stationery stores that were fronts for his numbers-running business. Kassell had paid for police protection, and his stationery stores would post a piece of white paper with a yellow bird on it to indicate to the beat police that they should look elsewhere to make busts.[29] Thus the letter of Fitzgerald's song alludes to paper from a stationery store, or a numbers policy purchased at one of Kassell's stationery stores for a mother, or another protector, perhaps Webb. The "little girlie" of Fitzgerald's song is "peck-peck-peckin,'" like a bird. The yellow bird sign in Kassell's stores signaled that white numbers runners, unlike Black numbers runners, received police protection—the very protection that Fitzgerald didn't receive when she was arrested and imprisoned.

Sending to one's mother a letter that is subsequently stolen reverberates with slavery and then Jim Crow legacies of broken maternal/child relationships. Additionally, one primary activity engaged by girls at Hudson was writing letters to their mothers, something Fitzgerald, whose mother had already died, would not have done. Another popular activity, but only enjoyed by the white girls at Hudson, was singing in the prison choir; even though staff at Hudson were aware of Fitzgerald's phenomenal singing voice, they forbade her from participating. Adding these two together, perhaps the song comments on the fact that, within the prison, white expression and biological lineages were encouraged while Black expression was forbidden.[30] Any and all of these, and probably more, are at play in this seemingly simple song.

By paying attention to this overlooked song, I emphasize that crip world-making materializes within aesthetics, cultural production, and nonnormative modes of living, working, and making. The state cripped Fitzgerald through its racial, pathologizing criminalization of impoverished young Black girls; the state hovered near Webb, always prepared to declare him its ward. Through song, performance, and band collectivity, Fitzgerald and Webb forged tactics that protected them from carceral settings. By recovering this denigrated song, I have sought to model the work the individual chapters of this book do—focusing on small-scale, minor, seemingly unimportant cultural productions to theorize alongside them the alternate models and aesthetics of care that they propose.

Chapter Summaries

Chapter 1 opens the book with a survey of psychiatry's postwar enthusiastic use of computers alongside its ongoing deployment of audiovisual media. I consider these in relation to the time's rights movements. Through televisual productions and nontheatrical films, the psy professions sought to recuperate psychiatric institutions' tarnished public image. Contemporaneous to this public relations campaign, the computer industries used industrial cinema to market their new products to medicine and psychiatry. The cinematic production of computers for psychiatry, emerging experiments with portable video in psychiatry, the computerization of psy-research videos, and the cinematic visions of shifts in institutionalization stabilized the discipline through psychiatric ways of screening. Increased federal funding for psychiatric technologies and media itself emerged from conjoined national logics aimed at controlling unruly populations.

The succeeding chapters explore alternate ways of screening produced by Black, feminist, and crip subjects. Chapter 2 examines computers and cinema at Lincoln Hospital Mental Health Services within the struggles for community control of Lincoln Hospital that extended from 1969 to 1971 and beyond. To the existing and ever-growing literature on these events, my analysis reveals that feminist-of-color critique articulated a politics of information activism to the radical politics developed and enacted by the multiple groups (the Young Lords, Lincoln Collective, and the Health Revolutionary Unity Movement) involved in these struggles. In chapter 3, I recover two Black-authored cultural works (a film and a television documentary) about mental distress made in the early 1970s. Situating these within the context of state-produced educational cinema and broadcast television documentaries about "the problems of the ghetto," chapter 3 foregrounds their challenges to the psychiatric gaze that pathologized communities of color. The media-technological production of racialized pathology occurred not only in state-sanctioned filmmaking but also through computer innovations produced out of the Cold War's cultures of simulation, the subject of chapter 4. I examine the development of the standardized patient in medicine and psychiatry, contemporaneous efforts to create computer simulations of psychiatric patients, and psychiatric "experiments" with live simulations. These offer new insights into psychiatry's use of technologies and media to exculpate it from accusations of racism. The chapter centers Black cultural productions that engaged with and critiqued simulation as a racializing and pathologizing way of screening.

The coda considers contemporary psychiatric digital media technologies. These cannot be understood as separate from our era's ongoing and increased antiracist and anti-ableist movements. A shiny new version of an old thing, the massive investment they spark reminds us of the value, today, generated out of governing the spillover.

Careful Language

As historians of psychiatry and Black disability studies scholars remind us in different ways, applying contemporary terminology to past historical moments is tricky business. This book is careful in its terminological choices for those entities variously named "mental health" and "mental illness." When I discuss people or states of being prior to or outside their capture by psy-entific discourse, I use terms such as "experiencing mental distress" and "experiencing addiction." Additionally, this book uses "the psy-ences" to refer to both disciplines of psychiatry and psychology. These are academic disciplines steeped in scientistic discourse, whose claim to those Western Enlightenment values of truth and objectivity this book takes as their hallucination. Perhaps they might be better called "psycho-ences."

1

PSYCHIATRIC WAYS OF
SCREENING IN THE LONG 1960S

In his 1967 presidential address to the American Psychopathological Association, Bernard Glueck Jr., director of the Institute of Living, a private psychiatric hospital in Hartford, Connecticut, exhorted the benefits of computers for psychiatry.[1] In the speech, published the next year as the lead editorial in a *Comprehensive Psychiatry* issue on automation and psychiatry, Glueck vividly portrays his perspective of America, in particular his imagined dangers threatening American society and American psychiatry. He cites fears that schizophrenics released from asylums are "poisoning" communities' "genetic stock." He notes the "insatiable demand" for psychiatric services "from the courts, prisons, schools, in fact from every segment of our society." He writes that in addition to society's insatiable demands on psychiatry, there is the insatiable demand for health and mental health care professionals' time created by information overload. In another article, Glueck framed the recent passage of Medicare—legislation passed in the wake of the rights movements—as overwhelming psychiatry with its indeterminant populations, with "future demands for accommodation by hospitals of an increasingly mobile population which will be highly dependent on computer-processed federal support programs."[2] Glueck concludes that these gargantuan appetites and dangers can be appeased by computers, in particular because they will allow experts to mine psy-entific datasets in order to select "fit" leaders for a society threatened by potential communists (and, by implication, queers). In sum, Glueck promoted computers through eugenic, Cold War, and racialized discourses. Computers were the bulwark against internal threats to and excessive demands on American society by those designated pathological—a bulwark that would also reinvigorate white male professional authority, propelling it to its appropriate position of authority in determining who was fit and who was unfit.[3]

It is not surprising that Glueck used the occasion of his presidential address to promote computers to his psychiatric peers. In addition to his assiduous efforts throughout the 1960s to incorporate different companies' computers into the Institute of Living, Glueck had also appeared in the IBM-produced film *Medical Information Systems* (ca. 1966), in which administrators and researchers at academic departments, medical hospitals, and, in Glueck's case, a private psychiatric hospital testified to the wonders of IBM systems. Whatever Glueck's significance (or insignificance) to the history of psychiatry, his work is emblematic of the crossover among the psychiatric industries and computer industries in this era, a crossover significant in securing the legitimacy of both. His discursive framing of computers as necessary for reestablishing psychiatry's authority to govern US society evidenced a revanchist response to the intense cultural, social, and political questioning of both computers and psychiatry. In Glueck's work, we see the concerted efforts required to normalize, justify, and legitimate the use of new computing technologies.[4]

This chapter argues that psychiatry took up technology and media in this period as part of its project of renewal. Directed at audiences uneasy with the opening of asylums and with increasing automation, films such as *Medical Information Systems* promised that psychiatry would be renewed through its engagement with computing and media. They were directed as well at professionals—both national authorities as well as local professionals—concerned about what Glueck glossed as the anticipation of an "insatiable demand" for psychiatric services by new patients. These "new patients" would be those covered under the recent passage of Medicare, one year after Title VI of the Civil Rights Act barred federal funding for any institution that practiced discrimination, and they were anticipated to be largely working class and of color. Glueck's "dreamwork" of automated psychiatry, then, arose out of anxieties over managing and medicating the "newly released schizophrenics poisoning genetic stock" as well as new populations—Black, Brown, working class—accessing psychiatric services, often involuntarily. In this chapter's readings of promotional media for computing, psychiatry, and the community mental health center movement, I illuminate how the intermediation of psychiatry and computers—which entangled federal agencies, psy-entific experts, authorities, and administrators, media and technology corporations, the broadcasting industries, and informatics industries—produced an assemblage of psychiatric ways of screening, which racialized as they pathologized. Psychiatric ways of screening both reflected the psy-ences' timorous cultural status and asserted their power to manage phantasmic irruptions to the social order. Taken together, the texts betray the psy-ences' deep anxiety over professional legitimacy, white male medical authority, and ongoing contestations to the disciplines' hold of the "spillover," that imagined specter of Black female sexuality and waywardness. Ultimately, these texts suggest a sublimation process that drove the intensified mediation and technologization of the psy-ences during this time.

The psy-entific media discussed here advanced racial pathologizing projects through their implicit coding of a psychiatry that was equipped with the latest media and technology as being able to flush out that spectral racial-pathological presumed to haunt and threaten the "American community." This psychiatric gaze was, by the late 1960s, being fervently contested by those whom it pathologized. Reading between the lines of data and documentation produced by the psy-ences, we can recover instances when what Autumn Womack names the violent racial data regime was challenged, if not refused.[5] By juxtaposing two experiments in participatory media-making within psychiatric contexts, I excavate a moment when young Black girls exposed psy-entific media and its data regime as a method of disciplining and silencing them. As with the segregated Progressive Era girls' prison examined in the introduction, a rehabilitation center visited by these girls, identified by the state as "at-risk" for delinquency, marshalled a racial pathologizing discourse that located the girls as "the spillover," as "adventurous thrill-seekers" whose presumed promiscuity threatened the social order. By exploiting the spillover they were presumed to represent, the girls used mediation to "un-discipline" the production of data. This chapter thus plumbs aesthetic and artistic engagements with and challenges to social scientific and positivistic epistemologies to read for buried contestations to the regulatory and disciplining work of psychiatric ways of screening.[6]

Computers in Psychiatry:
Administrative Control and Racialization

Throughout the 1960s, computing technologies buttressed racializing projects, whether in the United States, where law enforcement integrated computing into its racialized regime of violence and incarceration, or in South Africa, where apartheid depended on computer databases.[7] While computer companies made their technologies integral to these instruments of state violence, they also marketed their products to racial liberalist audiences, discursively framing them as appropriate instruments to address large-scale social problems. The 1965 CBS documentary *Watts: Riot or Revolt?* concluded with narration that referenced the Moynihan Report's diagnosis of "the Negro problem" as democracy's greatest dilemma; then, after the credits, one frame appeared and identified IBM as the film's sponsor. As Charlton McIlwain argues, the documentary's conclusion implied that IBM offered a remedy for America's "Negro problem."[8]

Computers were integral to community mental health centers from their very beginning, and their integration also originated out of the specter of unruly (and undeserving) populations. Prior to the passage of the Community Mental Health Act of 1963, through Title V demonstration grants the National Institute of Mental Health (NIMH) funded the introduction of IBM computers at a number of mental health institutions;[9] after the act passed in 1963, NIMH funded a growing number of sites' computer needs;[10] and by the late 1960s, computers were essential components of community mental health center grants, as they were necessary to ensure that centers could fulfill the act's mandate for evaluation and research. It is this mandate itself that enshrined that specter: Pentagon and other officials who crafted Great Society Initiatives were suspicious of social welfare programs, in part because of such programs' calls for democratic participation, which contradicted the officials' own ideological stances as well as their professional investment in models of centralization.[11] This underlying suspicion drove the federal government towards a systems analysis model that increased funding for policy research in the later 1960s and the early 1970s, a model that ultimately made computers and their data processing integral to social welfare programs that were required to evaluate whether federal policies, including those directed at impoverished communities of color, were effective. While care professionals sought to provide services to expanded communities and outside of a carceral system of institutionalization, those services would be beholden to a data regime that was legislated as mandatory.

Historians of computing argue that computing emerges not only due to legislative support but also due to multiple layers of production, consumption, and circulation (layers that are both explicitly and implicitly addressed through this book). Less explored in these accounts has been what Logan Brown calls a "media history of computing," which expands histories of computing by illuminating how computers were normalized via *useful cinema*.[12] In part because "mental hygiene" was a significant genre of useful cinema and in part because useful cinema widely circulated within mental health centers themselves, Brown's "media history of computing" is a productive frame for approaching the intersections of computers with media with psychiatry. As Brown documents, IBM was prolific in its production and circulation of useful films: they were loaned out through libraries and were exhibited at high schools, at colleges, and for adult audiences. IBM's useful cinema films were intended to stir interest in the understaffed profession of programming and to overcome cultural anxieties about automation. They would also counter visions of renegade cybernetic systems promulgated in science fiction films and elsewhere.

IBM's *Medical Information Systems* (1966) adroitly addressed such anxieties at the same time that it normalized computers in psychiatry and medicine. In this film, computing and informatics were linked to prestige, modernization, and mastery, links that recuperated white male authority through technologization. In *Medical Information Systems*, administrators at the nation's prestigious research and medical centers, including Glueck—who had been, two years prior to the film's production, working with IBM to develop psyentific programming languages for IBM computers at his Institute of Living— explained their facilities' use of computers. Accompanied by orchestral music in a major key, the film opens to full-screen text announcing the film as "A Motion Picture Report," text that echoes the newsreel reports shown before theatrical releases and that codes it as presenting of-the-moment information of national significance. Scrolling text identifying twelve esteemed research institutions appears over shots of nameplates and buildings, among them Johns Hopkins University School of Medicine, Harvard Medical School, Tulane University, the University of Texas Medical Branch, and University of California Los Angeles (UCLA), markers of academic institutional prestige and, through the sheer number of institutions, IBM's saturation of a market.[13] With no further introduction or framing narration, the first scene opens to an expert, identified by in-frame text as an authority at the Texas Medical Center, speaking from behind a desk. Wearing a white physician's coat, he discusses what he calls "the newest innovation in caring for patients": computerization. This white male personification of authority repeats through the film: each segment skips to different institutions, and all of their figureheads are white-seeming male administrators, clinical professors, and computing science librarians discussing how information systems are integrated into their facilities' operations.

Their discussion during this thirty-two-minute film can be best described as pedestrian, the banality of their words mirrored in the film's form, which uses static framing and includes little to no action in the mise-en-scène. Computing and information systems within hospitals would add rational, logical order, not drama and action; they were unlike countercultural representations of computers and Western technologies as mad (for example, in Ken Kesey's 1963 *One Flew Over the Cuckoo's Nest* and in Stanley Kubrick's 1969 blockbuster *2001*). Under the rubric of a "news report," the film directs the viewer's gaze to the relationships among men and machines and the orderly functioning of the offices, laboratories, and examining tables in the mise-en-scène.[14] Medical experts speak directly into the camera while sitting in bookshelf-lined offices, in armchairs before a fireplace, wearing physicians' white coats or business suits, smoking pipes in a classroom, writing with sterling silver or stainless steel pens, a fancy watch visible when a wrist cuff falls back. The semiotics of educational and institutional prestige and knowledge production permeate each scene.

As each man—and they are all men—describes the IBM technology used at his facility, the visuals cut from mid-shots of experts in office settings to close-ups of data visualizations on paper, or to women operating the technologies at, for example, a hospital admissions desk. These cuts demarcate conventionally gendered roles: Men are troped as knowledge producers without authorizing speech; women are silent laborers. While men speak directly facing into the camera, women are shown only with their eyes down, focused on their work. The film thus enacts this datafied gaze as an articulation of white male authority over knowledge production and the workplace.

Missing from the film are patients. A few scenes show people prior to or after hospitalizations—a couple with a blanketed baby at the admissions desk; a couple at discharge being handed a computer-generated bill. In three scenes, patients' bodies rest on examination tables, their faces never visible. In one instance, a clinical professor stands next to a patient on an examining table hooked up to a machine, yet the patient's head is cut out of the frame. This framing deliberately removes the patient as person from the scene; patients are merely props—bodies upon which technologies are operated by an expert seeking to produce knowledge. Traces of patients exist in pans over printouts of data, and in two shots it is possible, if one slows down the playback speed, to discern patients' names, but a person fully engaged as a subject within health care is absent. In scenes from Glueck Jr.'s Institute of Living, no patients appear, and tight shots on male researchers and female nurses effectively erase any depictions of care. Computers do not concern patients: They concern systems made more sophisticated and efficient. In this film, men speak, women work, and patients disappear into the computational realm of dot matrix printers and cathode-ray tube (CRT) screens.

One scene, an exterior shot, is unique to this film, where all other scenes are interior. After a close-up of the University of Missouri's engraved logo, a single-engine airplane lands on a field. An older white man, identified as the university's dean and director, leans against the airplane and discusses how computers will solve his profession's major crises: decreased numbers of family practice physicians, increased volume of information, and an increase in medical specializations. "[Computers]," he says, "make a wealth of information immediately accessible to the staff and students who must learn today to practice the medicine of tomorrow." The plane's side door remains open, so that visible behind the dean are the plane's dashboard, dials, and controls. Here, the visual cleaving of modern technology instantiated in the dashboard cockpit to the dean's triumphing of computers as modernizing bedraggled medical care joins elite male power to modernity, autonomy, and aerialism. The cockpit, as historians of this era argue, figured technological and cybernetic control, one in which the data flowing into a master controller allow it to modulate the system for efficiency and precision.[15]

The dean's figuration against the cockpit background does more than indicate cultural prestige, technological modernity, masculinized authority, and whiteness. It also ties this symbol of cybernetic control to his discussion of the crises facing medicine, suggesting that the "god's-eye view" of both the aerial pilot and the cybernetic controller allows separation from and control over the social. In 1966, the social was occupied with deeply contested discourses about how poverty and racism contributed to mental and health conditions. Specific to health and mental health care and academic medical centers, Medicare's passage had ensured the continued desegregation of hospitals— what Glueck described as creating an insatiable demand for psychiatric services.[16] It also helped force the continued desegregation of medical schools. As historians of medicine W. Michael Byrd and Linda Clayton put it, the Civil Rights Movement's successes, along with the passage of Medicare, forced white organized medicine to admit Black students to medical schools in the 1960s.[17] Speaking from a tarmac in a southern state, this dean's claims that computers are the "fix" to the shortage in general practitioners must be understood in light of what caused that shortage: medical racism, which, in the South, took the overt form of denying Black people entry to medical schools. Emphasizing the technological and eliding the social, the aerialist dean positions computers as a master controller that literally evacuates medicine of the social. The belief that modern technological systems enable the disappearing of the social/racial parallels the film's representation of technological medicine and psychiatry as white. IBM's medical information systems, the film proposes, will be used by white male organized medicine and its institutions to maintain white medicine's control over care.

A later promotional film, produced by IBM competitor Control Data Corporation, follows *Medical Information Systems'* administrative gaze of white medicine. Unlike IBM's film, *Early Warning* (McGraw Associates; ca. 1970) uses narrative and formal elements borrowed from feature filmmaking. In doing so, it demonstrates how computers' entry into health care enlisted cultural tropes, in this case, B-movie conventions that linked unruly physiological and mental states to systemic breakdowns. Like *Medical Information Systems*, *Early Warning* depicts both medical technologies (in heart care) and psychiatric technologies (the Minnesota Multiphasic Personality Inventory [MMPI]). Its opening, with its music and title style drawn from B-movie horror films, is distinctly different from IBM's film. Urgent, menacing music plays as a "Voice of God" narrator explains that computers are now being used in cardiac care. A sequence of titles appears: Large letters that almost fill the screen flash "EARLY WARNING!"; the next titles emerge in a small font that rapidly increases in size, stating "A Large Step for Medicine" and then "Improved Care for the Patient." As these three titles appear first over computer screens, then over surgeons operating at a table, the music's menace intensifies. A shift from the pedestrian managerialism of IBM's film, *Early Warning* uses B-movie music and titling to evoke anxiety about heart attacks and surgery.

This horror-inflected opening surgical scene transitions to the hospital's calm and orderly open office space, where nurses move among computers. Unlike in *Medical Information Systems*, in *Early Warning* nurses are identified by name and speak about computers, particularly how they have changed the way nurses work. The film grants nurses greater agency and authority than did *Medical Information Systems*; *Early Warning* identifies the multilayered forms of labor that computer and technological systems require. Ultimately, though, the film reproduces traditional gendered hierarchies of labor. The last quarter of the film discusses the MMPI, which its narrator explains contains questions a patient answers. "When scored, his answers may help diagnose any possible psychiatric disturbances and can offer some clue as [to] the origin of these disturbances." Subsequent scenes depict computers increasing the speed of processing MMPI data and analysis, and they highlight a white male programmer monitoring the punch-card reader. The narrator explains that the computer then produces a large report containing the information "in graph form, ready for the doctor in minutes." The film cuts to a doctor's office, in which a bespectacled older man looks over the report.

And while, like *Medical Information Systems*, this useful film mostly bores with its pedestrianism, in its coalescing of heart and psychiatric disturbances through the figure of an "early warning system," produced within the Cold War period and using elements from B-movies, the film positions computers as capable of identifying and managing disturbances "at the heart" of a smoothly functioning institution. Its setting—a Veterans Administration (VA) hospital—gestures to the military imaginary from which computers themselves arose, an imaginary of internal and external threats that computers could tamp out. Its final scenes of an American flag and a white man—at the film's start in a wheelchair, and now ambulatory—emphasize how computing technologies would renew American manhood.

Mediating Community Mental Health Centers:
Mental Health Films and Documentaries

While historians of psychiatry have understood the community mental health center (CMHC) movement as spurred by both the rights movements and by shifting paradigms in psychiatry itself, the role played in this history by the mediation of CMHCs has been underexplored. In 1949, soon after the National Institute of Mental Health was established, documentary and social realist filmmaker Irving Jacoby partnered with ten psychiatrists to form the Mental Health Film Board (MHFB). In its twenty-year life, the board produced more than fifty mental hygiene and mental health films, each in consultation with one or more board members, who included their day's most influential psy-professionals, including future and past presidents of the American Psychiatric Association. These films ranged in subject matter from family life, "troubled" adolescents, and old age to social work. Reviewed in psychiatric and counseling journals, the films, available for purchase or rental, were shown in diverse settings, including high school classrooms, community centers, and mental institutions themselves. Scholarship on nontheatrical public health cinema conceives it as biopolitical cinema—attempting to inculcate viewers into productive, self-managing citizenship.[18] Many MHFB film topics certainly fulfill these criteria; indeed, in a 1950 document announcing the MHFB's formation, Jacoby stated as much, writing, "The scope of the Mental Health Film Board is to . . . increase the productivity of the community by reducing the hidden forces that tend to make its members defeat their own purposes."[19] At least at its birth, the MHFB aligned itself with the biopolitics of the post-war psy-ences.

Before I explore the role that mediating CMHCs in the 1960s played in the longer historical arc of psychiatric ways of screening, I want to linger on an earlier MHFB production, an example that remarkably emphasizes the biopolitical reach of these films—in this case, a form of biopower. The 1953 MHFB-produced *Roots of Happiness* (dir. Henwar Rodakiewicz) was co-funded by the Puerto Rican Health Board and exhibited to Puerto Rican audiences as part of a US social science research study about population control methods. Social scientists who were connected to the influential Social Science Research Council used the film to study whether films or print pamphlets were more successful in persuading audiences to use birth control. This was part of what historian of empire Laura Briggs has argued was a colonial laboratory, one where Puerto Rico provided an experiment for US population control efforts designed to mitigate the fantasized communist threat posed by overpopulation: Puerto Rico was swamped with US social scientists, demographers, and economists taking as their focus "Puerto Rican reproduction and its responsiveness to family planning interventions," and the Puerto Rican mother's fertility in particular as subject.[20] The film, mostly narrated in English, took as its narrative two different Puerto Rican families, one with fewer children than the other, and focused on how to support Puerto Rican boys in their journey to "healthy" manhood; it also implied that having fewer children would result in greater household wealth. An outlier in the MHFB's productions, which more typically addressed middle-class white audiences, its production for social science research and use in US development efforts indicates that mental hygiene cinema was entangled in postwar geopolitical articulations of biopower.[21]

The mid- to late 1960s MHFB films mediating CMHCs promoted a vision of new forms of institutional care as bound to national renewal and a revitalization of psychiatry itself. Where postwar print, film, and sociological exposés such as *The Snakepit* (1948), Albert Deutsch's *The Shame of the States* (1948), and Erving Goffman's *Asylums* (1961) had revealed psychiatric institutions as horror shows, MHFB films conveyed psychiatry as in league with Great Society Initiatives renewing the American nation toward a more racially and economically egalitarian society. They worked alongside other useful film—including computer companies' marketing films—to link this renewal to other modernizing projects: research and computation. In these films, such modernization enabled psychiatric ways of screening populations.

One of many MHFB films produced to promote CMHCs, *Community Mental Health* (dir. Irving Lerner; 1967) employs a pedagogical narrative typical of MHFB films. While fictional, these pedagogical narratives aimed to demonstrate why and how communities should fund, plan, and build CMHCs. Often limited in narrative complexity and with spare production values, the films still drew from studio filmmaking; the opening scene of *Community Mental Health* does so, to surprising effect. Filmed in low light, shadows on a wall outline one human figure beating another, accompanied by nondiegetic music typical of 1960s film noir. This allusion to film noir continues into the next scene, when in voice-over a newspaper publisher recounts the incident of a young boy involved in a beating and theft. The narration by a newspaper worker, typical of film noir, also echoes the B-movie representation of asylums in *Shock Corridor* (dir. Samuel Fuller; 1963), which was narrated by its journalist protagonist, as well as the established genre of the newspaper film.[22] As the publisher explains in voice-over that he ran an editorial approving the trial's verdict of guilty for the boy, the film cuts to a scene more typical of melodrama: A group of four suburban white women drink coffee while heatedly discussing the event. The film shifts from the male voice-over to a voice-over from one of these women. She states that she and her neighbors thought the fight was propelled not by a lust for money but rather by something much deeper—"something that should have been noticed in him long before the crime was committed." They then discuss whether they might support increased funding for mental health services by applying for state funding. With the publisher's reluctant support, a committee is formed, town halls and fundraisers are held, and town members send to the state an application for funding for a CMHC, while the publisher explains that people will no longer be sent off to state facilities. The narrative resolves when the publisher reveals that the boy initially sentenced to trial will now be released and, in a narrative twist, that the boy is his own son.

Initially evoking film noir's perilous world and then ending with the comfort of familial and community resolution, the film's tonal tropes shift how MHFB films about CMHCs sought to redress popular shock-film representations of asylums, which had dampened public enthusiasm about psychiatry and related fields. The process of discovering the benefits of community mental health services dissolves noir's vision of a world of paranoia, pathologies, and criminality; a community-building effort oriented around "spotting the signs" before they evolve into pathologies interrupts, if not obviates, the dangerous horror of the asylum era. If noir in this era expressed Cold War paranoia, in *Community Mental Health* psychiatry and its services reconstituted small-town America as a bulwark against eruptions of pathologies, renewing communities through a collective effort to raise productive (white) citizens.

Other MHFB films about CMHCs illuminate that onto ideologies of national renewal such promotional efforts grafted psychiatric ways of screening. The 1966 film *Bold New Approach* (dir. Irving Jacoby) takes its title from President John F. Kennedy's 1963 speech announcing the Community Mental Health Act: "The time has come for a bold new approach" to mental health, he infamously stated. Presented by the NIMH, *Bold New Approach* visually and pedagogically illustrates the new facilities supported by the legislation. The film was widely exhibited at small showings hosted by city council agencies, mental health planning councils, and psychiatric hospitals themselves; it made it onto the Sunday television schedule for Scranton, Pennsylvania; and by 1970 it was one of many video cassettes available for rental through Sony's Electronic Video Recording system advertised for purchase by public libraries, its continued distribution a sign that it attracted interest as CMHCs spread.[23] In its careful attention to the architecture of CMHCs, the film supports other efforts to foster architects' and city planners' enthusiasm for such facilities. For example, writing in *Architectural Record* in 1963, the director of NIMH, Robert Felix, stated that the community mental health center "offers an exciting challenge to *American* architects, whose ingenuity and imagination will largely determine the shapes that these new edifices will take in the next few years" (emphasis added).[24] A few years later, in Houston, Texas, Rice University held an architecture conference showcasing responses to this challenge and published a two-volume report that included case studies, suggestions for the consultative process, and design checklists.

As a lesson in city planning and architecture, the film reflects a concerted effort to inspire professionals to redesign mental institutions to align with plans laid out in Great Society Initiatives, and it ties such redesigns to both *national* and *professional* renewal. The film opens to Stanley Yolles, the National Institutes of Health director, explaining the 1963 legislative act, with an intercut scene of President Lyndon Johnson signing the legislation. The film then moves into its fictional narrative, in which a town planning council member and an architect discuss the facilities needed to construct a CMHC in the fictional town of Foxington. These expository scenes in an interior office space are intercut with exterior and interior scenes from CMHCs that illustrate the kinds of activities, patients, staffing, and buildings their exposition describes. This shift from Yolles's direct-facing exposition in a formal office setting, which draws from the "talking-head" genre of mental health instructional media, to the discussion between two men within a modern office building, which narrativizes Yolles's explanation, formally indicates the film's themes of institutional transitions: Now-outdated mental institutions, like the traditional format of the "talking-head expert," will be modernized and made more approachable, a "discussion" between people rather than a dictate from a higher authority.

The film's credit sequence visually emphasizes the theme of modernization. As seen in figure 1.1, its title is superimposed over a midcentury modern metal sculpture hanging on a white wall, with a compositional style that mirrors feature films of the era. The camera cuts to the outer hallway of an office, where one wall bears a placard reading "Architects," and men carrying architectural plans enter and exit a doorway. The camera slowly tracks through the office space's open-plan configuration, revealing a long row of drafting tables where men hunch over their desks, working on plans. The film uses the straight angles of its mise-en-scène's architecture for compositional effect, in one instance dividing the credits across the vertical plane created by a wall (fig. 1.2), a compositional effect that again mirrors its era's feature films. When the credits end, with the director's name appearing over a close-up of a scale architectural plan (fig. 1.3), the camera continues to pan through the room until it rests on two men seated on a large couch. This opening credit sequence, leading the viewer from the exterior to the interior of an architecture firm, from built space to scale model, situates this "bold new approach" within the office bustling with male expertise.

The visual focus on the open-floor plan, on midcentury modern design, and on architecture as expert profession emphasizes the newer, midcentury understandings of architecture as available to all through the consumerist diffusion of mass-produced design objects.[25] As Lynn Spigel discusses in *TV by Design*, popular media in this era disseminated design culture from museums to the masses.[26] For Spigel, the use of cutting-edge graphic design by network television "taught viewers how to see [older forms of entertainment] within a modern context. . . . [M]odern graphic design reconfigured the old media for the new."[27] By invoking cutting-edge graphic design compositionally, and by including in the mise-en-scène markers of modern design, *Bold New Approach* visually connoted the new design of US psychiatry, whose "bold new

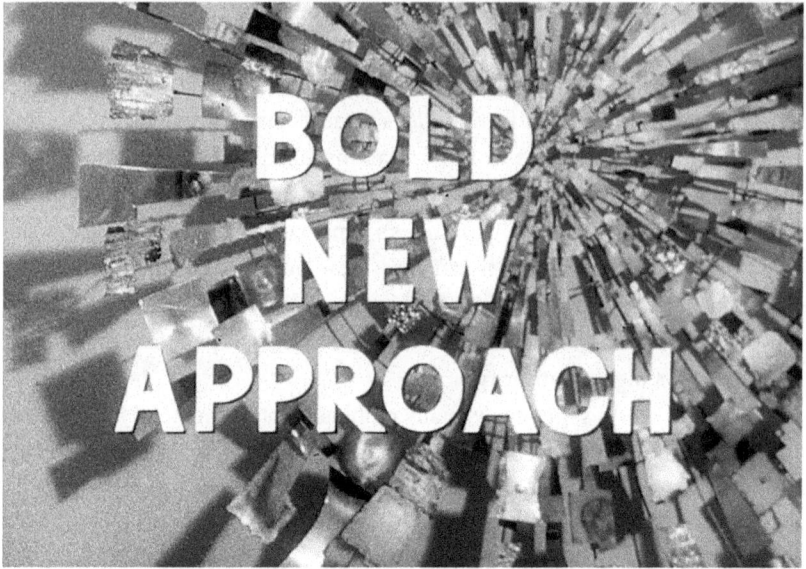

FIGURE 1.1. Title frame of *Bold New Approach.*

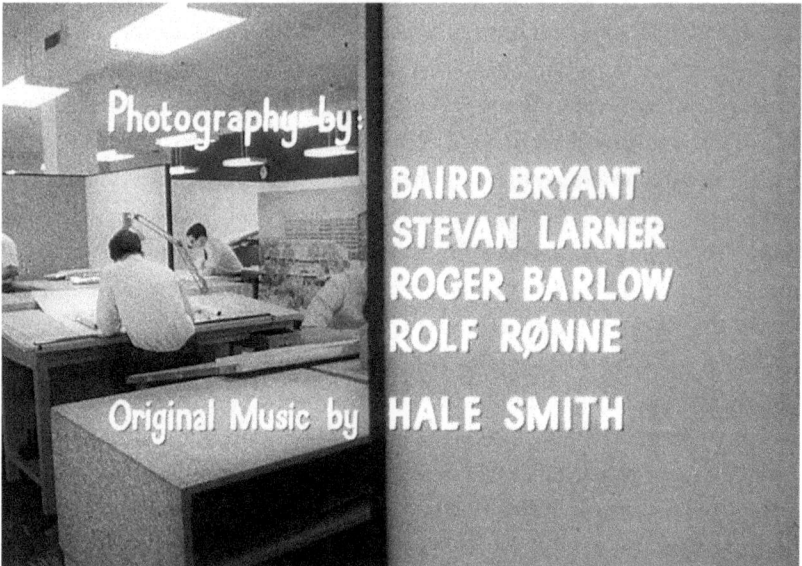

FIGURE 1.2. Credits for *Bold New Approach.*

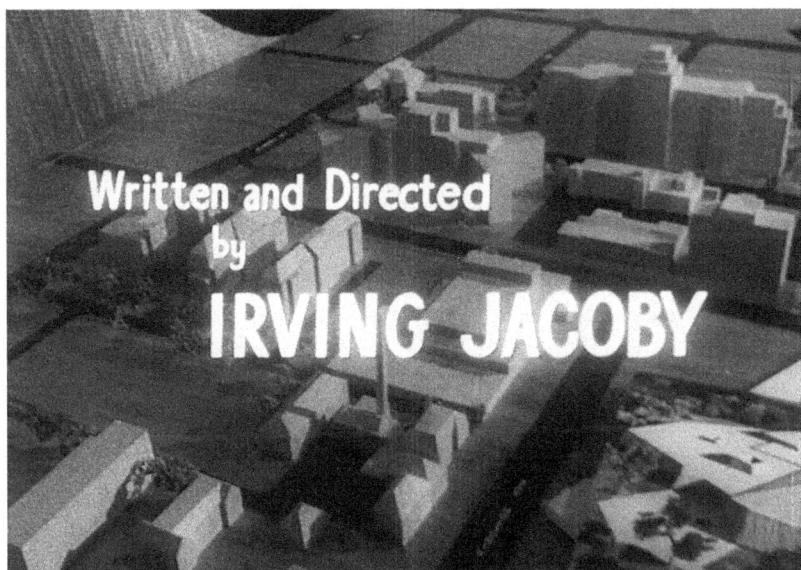

FIGURE 1.3. Director's credit, *Bold New Approach.*

approach" would modernize older psychiatric institutions now linked, in the public's mind, to questionable, if not horrific, practices.

As illustrated by figure 1.2, *Bold New Approach* employed a midcentury aesthetic of the grid. Perhaps most familiarly used in Alfred Hitchcock's title sequences of this era (for example in his 1959 *North by Northwest*), the grid and modular design moved into film style through the work of Saul Bass, who bridged both the corporate advertising and film industries; it was also popularized in the midcentury work of the Eameses.[28] But when implemented within a film about biopolitics, the grid is more than just the importation of visual tropes invoking "the modern." The grid is a cultural technique by which order is imposed and subjects are rendered into their proper places.[29] Here, the film's composition evokes the cultural logic of a grid, used by town planners, real estate industries, and architects. In essence, the film evoked the professional design of a CMHC as composing a town through the order and regularity of a grid imaginary: an organizational schema of control.

Modern design as modernizing psychiatry is realized as the two men visualize planning for a CMHC by building an architect's scale model on a large table. As the men build the scale model, the film cuts to scenes from existing CMHCs, providing "live" examples. The film uses as its example of ideal CMHC aesthetics a new European clinic. In this clinic, cozy rooms are built to serve a rotation of day and night patients, designed "to contribute to the closeness of the relations between these members of an institutional family." The segment on this clinic—indicated in one shot as Danish, even as the film's voice-over names it European—is the film's longest, and through the emphasis on a non-American clinic, it underscores that modern, European design can modernize *American* psychiatric institutions. Furthermore, its meeting rooms with entire walls of windows, wood-paneled interior walls blending the interior with the exterior, and light-filled rooms give it a distinctly "California" feel, an aesthetics of "easy living" also connected to midcentury design.

While "easy living" is seemingly contradictory to a grid imaginary, the emphasis on sight and visibility links the two. As the two men discuss where to locate a building designated for research, their voice-over narrates scenes of professionals of color driving through dilapidated city streets and gazing out car windows. These "explorers," the voice-over tells us, seek out new unserved communities, by implication applying a psychiatric gaze to what are troped as "urban slums." Suturing its scenes of research to scenes about impoverished communities of color, the film connects as-yet-unseen pathologies with racialized communities, yoking their eventual visibility to the data regime of research. Unlike its other segments on clinical services, the film spends little time showcasing a research building's interior; instead, the men decide to subtract the research building from their architectural model, stating that the local university's existing medical sciences center can house such research. The outreach that CMHCs would do into "slums" would be overseen by the modernizing project of the university.

In her work on the architecture of CMHCs, hospitals, and prisons during the Great Society years, Joy Knoblauch names the time's dominant architectural design model "psychological functionalism": "the use of form for its alleged emotional and behavioral impacts on occupants, [which would be] studied and implemented by a nation in search of new institutional forms to solve larger social problems of health, mental health, justice, and security of the population."[30] Certainly *Bold New Approach* illustrates that modernized CMHC architecture was conceived of as ameliorating the emotional and behavioral health of patients. The film also views such architecture as ameliorating the American town through transforming American professionals.[31] (As chapter 2 will show, the architectural design of one CMHC included in *Bold New Approach*— Lincoln Hospital Mental Health Services, located in the predominantly Puerto Rican area of the South Bronx—failed to live up to this functionalism, at least if we are to judge by the radical workers' takeover of the hospital just a few years after.) Toward the film's end, planning commission members—among them, a priest, a nurse, and a city welfare officer—view the architectural model and appreciate it as deepening their ability to provide care. The architect, who has spent his career building civic centers, expresses a newfound desire to focus on CMHCs. "But after all, community is people! And it would be the people of Foxington who would be treated in the [community mental health] center we were building. . . . Somehow through this job, I'd come closer to the community than I'd ever been before. I finally completed my education that afternoon." Renewing the town through modernizing its mental health services thus achieves a renewal of the professional expert's commitment to his profession and his town. This resolution holds an implicit appeal to the presumed expert professionals in its expected audiences: Building services for people designated pathological would renew, rather than destroy, the ethos of small-town America. Expert planning, guided by the organization of the grid, could rehabilitate the "community" and professional identity.[32]

While *Bold New Approach* glosses over the research center, the site of datafication, public television documentaries about these new psychiatric services engaged with computers for research as instruments of renewal.[33] Broadcast on US public television stations, the eight-episode series *To Save Tomorrow* featured transitional centers from around the country.[34] Its production evidences public television's goal of public affairs programming that could address cultural conversations about psychiatric institutions and alternatives to institutionalization. This goal was almost realized in the aborted showing of Frederick Wiseman's *Titticut Follies* (1967), which exposed the inhumane conditions at Massachusetts's Bridgewater State Mental Institution. WNET was about to contract with Wiseman to show the film on national public television when the Massachusetts state supreme court ruled that the film violated Bridgewater's patients' and guards' privacy, and it restricted the film's viewership to only mental health professionals. Although the television broadcast was scuttled, Wiseman's film did play at a few film festivals, and word of its chilling look at Bridgewater leaked out; that, plus the subsequent court battles over it, moved it into the national press, all the way to *Life* magazine.[35]

The episodes of *To Save Tomorrow* might then represent a response to the palimpsest left by Wiseman's obscured film. They showed psychiatric services and their patients in a destigmatizing light, with the explicit aim of fostering an appreciation for transitional housing and outpatient psychiatric services in apprehensive, NIMBY-ist communities. In particular, most episodes emphasized that those who in previous eras would have been locked away in institutions could be rehabilitated to fit capitalist norms of productivity.[36]

Formally, all eight shared an expository documentary style, in which either witness-participants provided extradiegetic voice-over or people in conversation were filmed to achieve a "fly-on-the-wall" feeling, accompanied by an unobtrusive musical theme. Each film granted the centers' male directors and psychiatrists the voice of authority, both through extradiegetic voice-over and through continually centering their on-screen explanations. In other words, psychiatric authority was once again gendered male.

Perhaps the strongest indication that the series aimed to rehabilitate the cultural reputation of psychiatric institutions lies in the unspoken links between the VA's Willow House, featured in *Operation Reentry*, and that cultural lodestar text of antipsychiatry sentiment, Kesey's *One Flew Over the Cuckoo's Nest*. In fact, Willow House was the very hospital at which Kesey had worked in the early 1960s and participated in LSD experiments, and he based his novel's depiction of mental hospitals on these experiences. *Operation Reentry* appears cognizant of this and of the cultural legacy of Kesey's character Nurse Ratched: It carefully showcases female nurses rehabilitating, rather than disciplining, the patients. As the director explains the token system used as a form of "operant conditioning" (rewarding for good behavior), he states, "The nurse and nursing assistants are able to manage the ward much more efficiently by asking the patients whether they want to earn tokens." The patients line up to exchange their tokens for items from the canteen, and one of them jokes with the dispensing nurse, who chuckles. Patients are also shown cleaning up the group meeting room, and the nurses, all Black women, hand out tokens to reward them for their good behavior. Ratched as a wielder of brutal control is replaced by nurturing Black nurses.

The episode about Fountain House, located two blocks from Times Square in New York City, takes the series into an urban locale known at the time for its strip clubs and peep shows. The episode opens to scenes that convey the area's entertainment, with 1960s go-go music as its theme. Walking through the area, the center's director, Dr. Beard, familiarizes viewers with an area that some might be primed to condemn as immoral. After he reaches the first Fountain House building, his narration about its history seems to situate this work as a renewal of a problem past. The film itself spends much of its narrative time showcasing its residents' job training. This includes scenes showing patients operating IBM punch-card machines, as in figure 1.4, where a white woman is shot from the side as she inputs data to a machine.

By privileging white patients as capable of rehabilitation, accompanied by these visions of technocratic order promised by the punch-card computer, the episode links independent living to productivity within and *for* the informat-

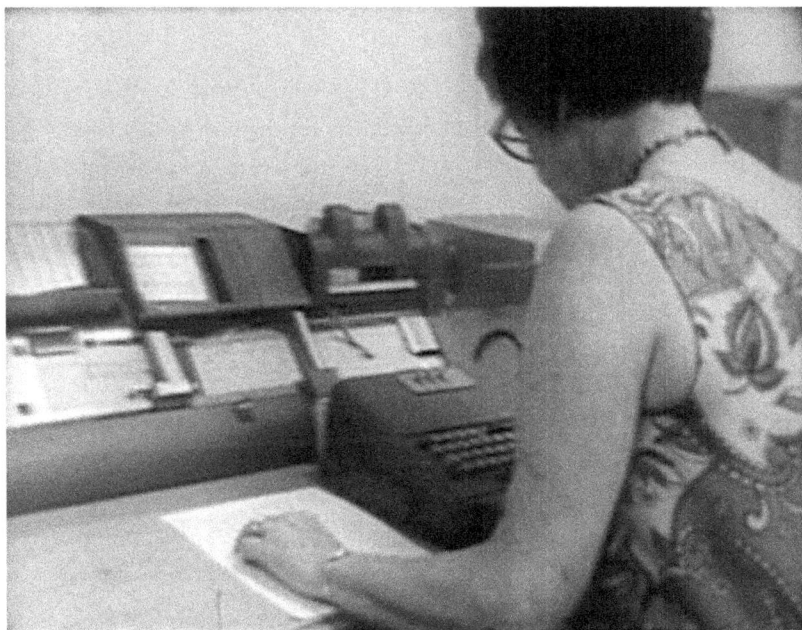

FIGURE 1.4. *Fountain House* (c. 1969).

ics industries. While Fountain House includes patients of multiple skin colors and, possibly, sexualities, the patients it shows at work, including working for informaticization, are all white.

In all of this, the irony of patients digitizing their own records of "madness" for research cannot escape the crip viewer. As much as large public institutions such as Rockland, so carefully illuminated by Jackie Orr, fostered the computerized governing of mentalities, community psychiatric formations, which claimed a distinctly different approach to mental health, similarly functioned as proving grounds for pathologizing technologies.[37] Mediating the CMHC movement as in step with a broader cultural push toward informatics, this episode assured viewers that control systems managed those designated pathologized. For IBM and its competitors, whatever cultural war was being waged over psychiatry, and where different institutions and their staff stood in this war, did not matter. What mattered was controlling the means of recording, and ultimately producing, pathologization.

Mediation, Cybernetic Systems, and
Countercultural Screens

This era's promotional efforts, instantiated in film and professional discourse, linked computers to a revitalization of medicine and psychiatry. As analyzed in the preceding sections, this theme of revitalization encoded a revitalization of white medicine and psychiatry's authority to govern an imagined threat to social order embodied by those populations that, after the passage of Medicare, would presumably overwhelm the professions. Whether at private psychiatric hospitals such as Glueck's or at publicly supported CMHCs, computers infiltrated the narrative imaginary of promotional and professional practices. During this era, alongside the computer industry the videotape industry also found willing innovators in the psy-ences, including two at Langley Porter Neuropsychiatric in San Francisco whose work would have lasting significance. Although quite different, in their similar media-technological genealogies they illustrate how psychiatric incarceration served research into systems of technologized control.

At Langley, Paul Ekman began this work in earnest, first, with 16mm film and, later, with videotape linked to computers.[38] Ekman is now widely known for his Facial Action Coding System, which underpins facial recognition and so-called emotional recognition technologies and which science and technology studies understands as a racializing assemblage of state and corporate carceral technologies.[39] Ekman's early work in a carceral psychiatric setting is one genealogy of this assemblage. In the late 1960s, Ekman's work was funded by the US military's Defense Advanced Research Projects Agency (DARPA), which supported researchers in developing technologies for imperial use and asserted the military usefulness of lie detection technology that interpreted facial expressions. Ekman used videotapes of Langley patients to develop a coding system for videotape, which he called the Visual Information Display and Retrieval (VID-R) system. The system linked two videotape recorders to a video recorder, a film-to-video "chain"; human operators would watch the videorecording and type into a computer the coded terms for what they saw. By building this index of terms, the system would make it much more manageable to retrieve specific moments of human interactions from vast archives of film and videotape. At the time, Ekman described the system's primary uses to be research into behavior, archival management, and student training. As discussed in the introduction, the origins of a current racializing and pathologizing surveillance technology within a carceral psychiatric setting indicates the centrality of psychiatric incarceration for media technological innovation.

In his published work on this system, Ekman does not indicate which videotapes or films he used, nor which incarcerated patients were videotaped. Thus, it is impossible to know whether Ekman produced new videotapes of patients or used existing videotapes made by other researchers, and it is not known which patients appeared in these videotapes. It is not surprising these details were elided: The purpose of the research was solely to validate the media technological method itself, and thus the patient was an irrelevant detail. It is possible Ekman used the voluminous videotapes already recorded at Langley Porter by Harry Wilmer, Langley's head psychiatrist. Even if Ekman didn't, Ekman's work—supported, in the 1970s, by the CIA, and in some senses therefore ideologically orthogonal to the liberal humanist and seemingly countercultural-friendly work of Wilmer—shares with Wilmer's a model of humans as integrated nodes within a cybernetic system.

In Langley's ward for young people who had used drugs, Wilmer researched videotape as a therapeutic modality. For Wilmer, by filming patients and allowing them to replay these recordings, videotape allowed a patient to see how others saw them. In so doing, the patient could recognize and reenter the system of human interrelations that Wilmer saw as key to successful therapeutic treatment. While Wilmer published about two separate experiments with videotape feedback—one at Langley, the other at San Quentin Prison—the documentary that Wilmer ultimately produced about his research, *Youth Drug Ward* (1970), showcased only his work at Langley.[40] Wilmer's documentary entered a cultural sphere replete with studio films about psychiatry. Summarizing studio films that depicted psychiatry, Michael DeAngelis argues that they recuperated any radical energies of new forms of group therapy, which emphasized "socio-political forms of connection," by grafting these onto "the one-on-one analyst/analysand model of psychoanalysis," thus retreating away from sociopolitical forms of connection for the individualized focus of the psychoanalytic couch.[41] Wilmer makes clear that he views group therapy conducted with videotape replay as restoring a more authentic (for patients designated addicts, more sober) form of sociopolitical engagement to his patients, and thus he appears engaged with newer forms of sociopolitical connective therapy. However, the documentary's depiction of traditional Freudian frameworks, as well as its formal embodiment of a Lacanian patriarchal symbolic, aligns the documentary with the conservative energies of studio filmmaking's representation of psychotherapy. That the documentary elides Wilmer's other videotape-replay experiment at San Quentin highlights not only the exigencies of documentary produced for public television—that it should straddle both white bourgeois taste cultures and more innovative fare—but also a repression involved in producing a free white subject that is worthy of rehabilitation via media.[42]

Wilmer, a Jungian psychotherapist with a background treating soldiers, had previous television experience. The ABC primetime television series *Alcoa Premier* featured Wilmer's work in its 1961 inaugural episode. Titled "People Need People" and narrated by Fred Astaire, the episode dramatized Wilmer's 1950s experiment in an Oakland, California, psychiatric facility, when he allowed World War II veterans confined there to live communally.[43] In the late 1960s, serving as the chief psychiatrist at Langley Porter Neuropsychiatric Institute, Wilmer opened a ward for what he, like many other liberal humanists of the time, called "mixed-up kids"—the hippies of Haight-Ashbury. In this ward, Wilmer used the portable recording devices that were being increasingly marketed outside the entertainment industry: There were videotape recorders, a 16mm film camera, an 8mm film camera, and audiotape recorders; the ward was also outfitted with a closed-circuit television system, already in use in prisons and mental institutions more broadly.[44] Even more impressively, as documented by Carmine Grimaldi, the institution had access to the University of California at San Francisco (UCSF) television studio and the seven staff members who operated it.[45]

While the documentary's aesthetics generally draw on cinéma verité, its opening moments evoke a more experimental style. Its first image is of what may be a television; on it displays a distorted image of a woman. This cuts to an image of a young woman—perhaps the one from the distorted image—who looks off-screen. Then the original distorted image appears again. Over these images, a man's voice states, "So the main reason we're here today is to watch the video, to see what we can learn from it. Let's watch the replay." While three title clips slowly appear—which give credit to the California Department of Mental Hygiene, Langley Porter Neuropsychiatric, and the UCSF School of Medicine—the man's voice narrates that, at Langley, cameras were used so that the staff could learn from the patients and so that residents could also learn from rewatching videotapes of their interactions with patients. The next sequence shows a young woman, seated in a leather easy chair, speaking toward the camera; in front of her, trained on and filming her, is another camera, which, in its viewfinder, displays the scene being filmed. She is at ease, draping herself over the chair, barefoot, and she describes how she no longer uses speed and is on a diet. Next, the film cuts to a group therapy scene, where the camera is at first focused on another young woman, who responds to questions from a voice off-camera, the same voice from the introductions.

From the start, then, the film draws on two aesthetic lineages: the first, experimental video practices; the second, cinéma verité. The experimental video lineage is not surprising, given that Wilmer eventually published on the youth drug ward in *Radical Software*, a zine that also included essays by practitioners of experimental video.[46] Videotape feedback as a process was already imbued with its experimental video art context. And while rough shots and cuts, moments of the subjects staring into the camera, and other formal qualities that explore the filmic apparatus draw on cinéma verité, it would be going too far to say that the film is explicitly cinéma verité. Rather, it uses certain cinéma verité conventions to make the filming and the ward seem as unchanged by its mediation as possible. By drawing on cinéma verité conventions, Wilmer's film conveyed the ward using one of the more radically coded documentary styles of the era. For the general American public, the lack of continuity and suture surely suggested that the content itself was edgy, not constrained by Hollywood conventions.

Over another montage of images of San Francisco, Langley Neuropsychiatric, and his patients at rest and at play, Wilmer explains why he decided to use videotape feedback in the ward. In 1967 the ward was opened specifically to serve hippies who, coming to the flower power streets of Haight-Ashbury, were having bad trips. As Wilmer put it, they were "adolescents on dangerous drugs, not hard narcotics" and the "therapeutic community" would be "aided by the electronic media." Wilmer went on to say, "The media, I feel, have been responsible for a great deal of the destruction of what was good in the hippies, what was hopeful in Haight-Ashbury, in the very beginning, in the flower culture. They were exploited in the media—television, film, press—but particularly, television. This was the first television generation . . . and it had inhibited them, made them passive people." After touching on the images of war and violence, particularly of Vietnam, that suffused media in the late 1960s, Wilmer concludes, "What was . . . frightening and overwhelming I thought contained in it healing qualities." Thus Wilmer justified for a national TV audience that the television apparatus could itself be used to heal the very harms it was causing. In this, Wilmer seemed to feed the kind of disciplining of television that Laurie Ouellette has identified occurring with the birth of public television.

Existing scholarship on Wilmer's videotape feedback considers it to be a radical experiment in cybernetic subjectivity, contextualizing Wilmer's work within a broader array of media experiments happening in the time period.[47] None of this scholarship has lingered, however, on what was not at all experimental about Wilmer's film: its conventional structuring through a patriarchal symbolic. This is all the more interesting in light of the fact that while Wilmer claimed to be experimenting within psychiatry, still he reinstituted the very symbolic that imbued the psy-ences. Much of the film embodies classical Hollywood cinema's male gaze. In fact, that opening montage of distortion, resolution, and distortion again is a canny, abstract instantiation of the Lacanian symbolic, a bizarrely apt lack followed by fulfillment followed by lack, as those poles revolve around the female figure as the object of desire in the male gaze. These beginning images of female patients are overlaid by a male voice explaining to the viewer the purpose of Langley and its cameras, and the very opening words are an imperative to "watch the replay," thereby constructing the voice of authority as masculine. That we will quickly discover the voice of authority is, here, the older male therapist seems to remarkably narrativize Freudian frameworks; this structures the entire film's treatment of therapy, no matter how "radical" for the time it might be, within a traditional patriarchal model.

The traditional patriarchal symbolic recurs in scenes showing video feedback's other application: training the residents on the ward. In voice-over, Wilmer explains that residents have conflicts. "The conflict of the resident is pretty specific. There's a need to relate intimately in the sense that it's honest, spontaneous, not hiding behind words or a professional cloak. . . . [In an unconventional ward like this,] he's lost his sense of identity, his role isn't clear—the nurse may have opinions about drugs and she feels she has a right to talk about it." The gendered nature of occupational positions within the ward is unmistakable here: The male residents are training to become therapists and to assert themselves when challenged by those beneath them in the occupational hierarchy. The one scene that focuses on the residents' conflict happens just after a group therapy session in which a young woman expresses her sexual desire for the resident leading the session. Afterward, the resident debriefs with Wilmer, where they discuss transference and how to work through it. Thus, the one expression of female desire (rather than the objectification of the woman) is quickly recontained within a narrative about how the male resident will resolve his desire. This indicates the resolutely patriarchal framework underlying the imaginary innovative moment of videotape feedback therapy.

Wilmer also framed his work in relation to the budding movement of participatory media production. For Wilmer, allowing patients to operate the cameras fulfilled a therapeutic function. *Youth Drug Ward* only ever shows male patients operating the camera. When we see nonidentified camera operators (probably members of the ward's staff), they too are male. In this, the film itself appears to masculinize media production, another instance wherein the documentary articulates conventionally gendered models of creative production and authority. Additionally, the three patients the film focuses on are white (two women and one man). This is not to say that there weren't patients of color on the ward—at one point as the camera moves through the ward, we see a Black woman, who gestures at the camera and appears to speak, but her words are silenced by the voice-over that never names her presence. In Wilmer's mediation of therapeutic participatory media, only white men appear as participants. The racial and gender differences that the Black woman represents put too much pressure on Wilmer's research framework and its mediation for the American public.

Participatory Psy Media and the Spillover

Wilmer's psy-entific media experiments at Langley cleaved together the psy-ences' move to incorporate videotape into treatment and therapy as well as a broader cultural trend of participatory media. Both these trends shared a rehabilitative logic. For the psy-ences, participatory media rehabilitated the individual patient. For some independent filmmakers, participatory media rehabilitated the sphere of cultural production away from its white elitism, for example through the Young Filmmaker's Foundation in New York; for others, participatory media rehabilitated youth of color, who supposedly had an impoverished expressiveness due to their so-called culture of poverty, which was theorized as stunting the development of young children of color.[48] The history of children's media experiments in the late 1960s and early 1970s has been richly documented both in scholarship and by those who implemented it, such as DeeDee Halleck.[49] For her part, Halleck viewed participatory media production less within a "rehabilitative" model and more as a mode for children from communities that an elitist white cultural sphere abjured to find voice and vision. While teachers such as Halleck instructed young people how to make movies, those working within the "culture of poverty" framework collected data about youths' media-making, subjecting it to the scrutiny of the data regime.

One such project, in which young Black girls' media-making was observed, studied, and coded into data by researchers, occurred circa 1969 at the Philadelphia Child Guidance Clinic. In their article about this project, the researchers justify researching youth media production within the framework of the "culture of poverty" thesis: "For a disadvantaged population that may lack verbal skills, film can be a means to express their view of the situation."[50] These two male investigators met with girls ranging in age from twelve to fourteen, plus a sixteen-year-old girl who later joined them, to establish the project's contours: The investigators would provide technical assistance and a schedule for film production, with no influence whatsoever on the film's content. "In return," they wrote, "[we] would do [our] researching, recording and observing of the girls as they went about making their film. *That was the contract*" [emphasis added].[51] The girls thus expressly understood that their aesthetic production would be fodder for a regime of data. And, so, it is not surprising when next the investigators complain that production was slowed because the girls were more interested in being actresses than film producers. After all, what research subjects would not want to cloak themselves in the signifying possibilities of performance? For the investigators, this issue in efficient filmmaking was superseded by "the girls' inability to function as a group and to solve their organizational problems."[52] Here we see the essence of this study: collective cultural production as figurative of sociality, or, in other words, the investigators' aim to study "group organization" via media-making.

In this film's archival absence, I rely on reading against the grain and between the lines of the investigators' report. Here is how they describe the film that the girls produced. A young mother, Carolyn, lives with her baby and her own mother. After her mother derides Carolyn's mothering skills and tells her to give the baby up for adoption so Carolyn can "run the street with those wild girls," the daughter slaps her, and the mother throws her out of the house. Carolyn moves in with her girlfriends, who share an apartment with a few boys. In the next scene, the residents celebrate with some drinks, leading to a drunken fight among them all, except for one, who laughs while watching them. The investigators relate that, after a few more weeks, the girls wrote the next part of the script, a scene in which their film's female characters leave to obtain marijuana but are caught up in a police raid, Carolyn is imprisoned, and, finally, the police raid the apartment, imprisoning all the girls and giving Carolyn's mother her baby. Unable to cast actual police and film this particular part, the girls rewrote the final scene: They wrote on a blackboard an intertitle, "The Cops came and arrested the girls." Then, a substitute final scene was created in which Carolyn lies drunk on a couch, and her mother knocks on the door. She enters and takes Carolyn's baby away, after which Carolyn states, "Free at last, free at last, fuck that bitch, I'm free at last." This concluding line did not make it into the final cut of the film. According to the investigators, "several weeks later, after deciding the film's sound recording was not adequate for reproduction purposes, the investigators asked the girls to re-record [this final scene's] dialogue as they watched the film's workprint."[53] In the final cut of the film, Carolyn did not speak; rather, she silently followed the mother, who had come for her baby, out the door.

Was the spoken obscenity too much for the investigators? Or did it have to be elided because it signified on the final lines of Martin Luther King Jr.'s "I Have a Dream" speech in a manner that some racial liberals might find concerning? Close reading reveals that while the investigators wrote that they only desired re-recorded dialogue, in actuality they removed dialogue and silenced Carolyn. The girls' desired final ending was, therefore, elided through the investigators' active intervention—an intervention they had "contracted" not to do. Let me put this a bit differently. In their original vision, the girls verbalized "Free at last, free at least, fuck that bitch, I'm free at last," substituting MLK's "thank god almighty" with a different articulation of the conditions for Black girls' liberation—one in which they consciously severed bonds with their mothers, or with the maternal, or with the forces insisting they inhabit the proper maternal role expected of a properly rehabilitated woman. Perhaps this was a rejection of the ongoing failure of racial liberalism to liberate them, and a knowingness that racial liberalism's aim was to recontain them within tropes of the proper maternal figure. It would seem then that the revised ending inserted the investigators' recontainment: the Black girl muted within the now-reinstated figuration of the maternal.

Even after the filmmakers revised the film's original ending, its existence caused a "crisis" within the clinic. The researchers noted that one Black community organizer told them "riots start over things like this," and other Black community workers, among them Black Panthers, upset that the film reveled in depicting Black life through stereotypes of pathological behavior and suspicious that the investigators themselves had shaped the film, demanded that the film be destroyed. The investigators pushed back, arguing that the girls had decided the film's content and it should be up to the girls to decide the film's fate. Indeed, in her work, Deborah Weinstein argues that the controversy the girls' film provoked among all levels of staff at the clinic and its community workers "implicated the politically charged relations between a clinical institution and its surrounding community."[54] And yet the investigators' related participatory media experiments with other youth groups— impoverished Black male youths, impoverished white youth, middle-class Black youth, and middle-class white youth—did not provoke any similar controversy; at least, if they did, the projects' investigators did not document it as they did the controversy over the girls' film. Why, then, the girls?[55]

Here, I want to discuss this incident in relation to what Jonathan Metzl describes as the deafening silence about Black women's experience of psychiatric incarceration in this era.[56] As Ayesha Hardison argues, such silences are due to the epistemic injustice of racist misogyny, which has no heuristic by which to comprehend what has been spoken.[57] Epistemic justice might be done to this presumed silence if we read this moment of girls' media production, meant to serve the racial data regime, differently than its researchers read it. Emphasizing that they offered the girls "a contract," we might ask whether, in this situation of unequal power relations, the girls were in any position to give informed consent. From minor details the researchers include, the girls were testing the terms of this contract. They annoyed the researchers by playing around as actresses, refusing to fulfill the contract's mandate that they produce the film. They irritated the researchers by continually testing whether the researchers would hold up their (contracted) bargain that they would not influence the film's content. They ground up the researchers' desire to "study group dynamics" by conflicting with each other and pursuing other activities they found to be more engaging. Minor annoyances for the researchers, the girls' flexes against the contract embody what we might call an instance of "informed refusal," a concept Ruha Benjamin offers in opposition to bioethics' "informed consent."[58] Although not articulated as such, their disruption of the study's procedures embodied an implicit refusal of the terms under which they had been "contracted."

It might be read as a moment in which black sociality, to draw from Autumn Womack, exceeded the disciplining context of its study.[59] Produced within the disciplining confines of a social service agency born of midcentury discourses of juvenile delinquency, guided through its nine-month (!) production period by well-meaning liberal media-makers who observed and documented the entire production process, and requiring that its subjects also document their process, the project entered the ongoing effort to quantify Black life—in this case, that of Black girls. That it nominally depended on the girls participating in artistic production means it must be read with attention to the friction its subjects, purportedly delinquent Black girls, introduced into this data regime.

Whether they intended to or not, the girls' media-making threw into disarray an institution whose mission advanced the regime of racial pathologization via documentation and data. The mental health clinic positioned Black girls within the disciplining force of discourses of hypersexuality, unfit mothering, and delinquency. Their representational reproduction of these modes of living—the very ones from which the clinic purported to "rescue" them—within a rigorously documented process exploded, via excess, the media and documentation of Black girls as a problem. To draw on La Marr Jurelle

Bruce, they tactically inhabited discourses of Black girls' pathology: They flexed "the spillover" to throw an institution of pathologization into disarray.[60] Indeed, one possible ending to the film—one of the scripts' coauthors told the investigators "and then everyone dies!" was the ending she desired—indicates the girls' knowledge that the continued reproduction of discourses of Black female pathology was a teleology of nonfuturity, a place of (social) death. In re-representing for this regime of disciplining data its own representations, the girls exceeded its logic, exposing the right to the psychiatric screen as an incitement to discipline.

Next, chapter 2 unearths another woman-of-color interruption of the regimes of racializing data that shaped psychiatric ways of screening within the move to community mental health centers. In the case of Lincoln Hospital, this interruption formed not through tactical inhabitation but rather strategic occupation. Women of color developed a feminist-of-color disability analytic that understood, and targeted for dismantling, the racialized data regime of systems of madness that debilitated communities of color.

2

FEMINIST-OF-COLOR ACTIVISM
AND INFORMATION JUSTICE AT
LINCOLN HOSPITAL

From 1969 to 1971, Lincoln Hospital in the South Bronx was a site of radical struggle. The protests and direct actions of workers and community organizers are now canonical within studies of solidarity movements, health activist histories, and feminist studies. They have been richly documented both through participants' retrospective writings (for example, Iris Morales's collection *Through the Eyes of Rebel Women*) and in such exhaustive histories of the Young Lords as Johanna Fernández's *The Young Lords: A Radical History*.[1] The documentary *Takeover* (dir. Emma Francis-Snyder; 2021) made adamantly clear the events' relevance to our own era of racialized health systems, of health workers' struggles for better wages and working conditions, and of the centrality of feminists of color to these struggles.

This chapter revisits these events, rereads their archives, and recovers a little-known film to make two arguments. First, these struggles included struggles over hospital information systems—an infrastructure that sustained what the era's activists named the "health empire"—and over hospital media. Second, feminists of color engaged in what we would now call "information activism." Although they did not use the term "information activism," review-

ing their struggle through this more recent formulation introduces new avenues of thinking crip genealogies in relation to the seemingly drab topic
of information systems.[2] Here, I open up new possibilities for considering
feminist-of-color thought as challenging systems of informatics that, in the
late 1960s, were not widely targeted for dismantling.

Feminist-of-color activists at Lincoln Hospital offered a key instance of
Sami Schalk and Jina Kim's feminist-of-color disability analytic, as they sought
community control of a resource-deprived hospital and its structural abandonment of Black and Brown populations.[3] For the feminists of color involved
in struggles at Lincoln Hospital, racialized resource deprivation was articulated to a politics of reproductive justice as well as a feminist-of-color politics
of information systems. Like the Young Lords and the Lincoln Collective—
a group of new left physicians and psychiatrists at Lincoln—feminists of
color viewed Lincoln Hospital as part of the health empire. This empire was
sustained to profit institutions of white wealth, including real estate corporations, insurance industries, academic research, and monied hospitals. Feminists of color brought the Young Lords' analysis of US empire to bear on this
health empire, viewing this resource deprivation as connected to reproductive injustices on the island of Puerto Rico, as well as on the US continent.
Over the course of two years of intense struggles to gain community control of
Lincoln Hospital, these women instituted information activism tactics. These
tactics were sometimes explicit interventions in health empire information
systems and health empire media. Sometimes these tactics were the indirect
outcome of the influence of feminist-of-color critique on other collectives,
including the radical filmmaking collective Newsreel. In other words, out of
feminist-of-color critique arose a sustained challenge to the media and technologies of a health empire that profited from screens that reproduced racial
pathologization and reproductive injustices. In what follows, I build this argument by discussing Lincoln Hospital Mental Health Services' educational
films, computers and information activism at Lincoln Hospital, and then a
little-known Newsreel documentary about the struggle for community control of mental health care.

Health Empire Media

In the Great Society Initiatives oriented around a "bold new approach" to
mental health, data quickly moved to the foreground. In 1963, the Community Mental Health Act was signed into law. In 1965, Great Society Initiatives, including the passage of Medicare and the establishing of the Office

of Economic Opportunity (OEO), provided new funding that would support community mental health services. In New York City, the "affiliation plan" partnered established and wealthy teaching hospitals with other local hospitals that served communities of color. The endeavors that these initiatives funded came to focus just as much on data gathering and research capacities as on clinical services.

Located in the predominantly Puerto Rican and Black neighborhood of the South Bronx, Lincoln Hospital was so run-down and understaffed that local residents referred to it as "the butcher shop" and, later, as a "slaughterhouse." The 1961 passage of legislation to place New York City's overtaxed municipal hospitals under administrative control of the city's private medical centers partnered Lincoln Hospital with the Albert Einstein College of Medicine at Yeshiva University. Drawing on federal funds made available through Great Society Initiatives, psychiatrists at Albert Einstein initiated Lincoln Hospital's first psychiatric services, a community mental health center named Lincoln Hospital Mental Health Services (LHMHS). The service spanned multiple locations: Local storefronts housed walk-in services, and Lincoln Hospital established dedicated space for in-patient and out-patient treatment. In line with Great Society funding that called for training impoverished people for specific professions, LHMHS encouraged neighborhood residents ("indigenous workers") to apply, and by 1966, LHMHS employed fifty-four Puerto Rican and Black residents of South Bronx as community mental health workers.

In their 1968 report about LHMHS prepared for the National Institute of Mental Health (NIMH), directors Harris Peck and Elmer Struening explained their training program for nonprofessional mental health workers. During their training, Puerto Rican and Black employees viewed two films that "show[ed] life in the slums of South Bronx."[4] One of these films, *Uptown*, may not have had its intended effect among the trainees: Peck and Struening report that one woman said she didn't know she was poor until she entered the program and that stereotypes such as "the poor are anti-education" or "the poor buy impulsively"—stereotypes articulated in *Uptown*—weren't accurate. Perhaps, she said, she wasn't poor at all. That film, directed by independent filmmaker Herbert Danska, veered from the day's dominant racial liberalist documentary practice, which aimed to spur white people's empathy for communities of color.[5] One such documentary, 1963's *Manhattan Battleground* (dir. William Jersey), follows a white social worker who lives among the Puerto Rican community in Spanish Harlem.[6] A middle-class heterosexed professional temporarily living in "the ghetto"—he leaves for medical school after his internship "in the field" is over—the social worker's abbreviated stay embodies a white liberal, middle-class intervention into settings of urban poverty. While this particular documentary centers on the emotions of both the social worker and those Puerto Ricans he works with, the film's conclusion highlights only the white social worker's emotional changes, those affective transformations wrought by his work with the community. This racial liberalist framing of urban poverty and social work—that helping a community of color *affects* individual white people—embodies the racial liberal imagination shaping documentary mediations of the well-being of the so-called inner city.[7]

Rather than working to elicit empathy in white viewers, in what I will refer to as a pedagogical mode, *Uptown* works to trouble dominant cultural stereotypes about the South Bronx. Nevertheless, just as empathy narratives objectify the people for whom empathy is being inspired and also re-create the very distance they aim to overcome, *Uptown*'s pedagogical narrative, which addresses an implied white, nonworking-class viewer, also produces a distancing effect. In so doing, it reinscribes a racializing mode of viewership.

The film begins with a black screen; across its bottom third runs, from right to left, a ticker-tape flow of all-capitalized words in newspaper-style font. Accompanying this ticker tape play the sounds of city streets: car horns, muted voices chattering. The ticker tape provides data on unemployment, the use of Aid to Dependent Children, juvenile delinquency, and youth venereal disease in New York City and in the South Bronx. In all these categories, rates for the South Bronx are higher. Then, the ticker tape lists homicide and suicide rates for Central Harlem and the South Bronx; homicide rates in Central Harlem are higher, while suicide rates in the South Bronx are higher. Finally, it gives a number of approximate psychiatric hospitalizations per month in the South Bronx. Absent a narrator, the data construct a narrative that implicates Central Harlem with violence and the South Bronx with pathologies.

The opening visuals are shots of airplanes and city roofs and of young men and women playing on the roofs, flying kites and balancing on walls. A gentle male voice says, "Here, outsiders say there's nothing much to see, nothing at all." The voice falls silent, and the visuals of roofs, birds, and kites fill the screen; the ensuing silence lasts longer than in a conventional documentary. This slow and contemplative temporality and affective tone give the viewer time to pause and concentrate. With the camera's slow movement across the bulky buildings' rooftops and its focus on the kite and birds aloft, the film's aesthetics verge on the lyrical.[8]

The narrator speaks again. "We've seen this elsewhere, in other cities, so much that we no longer realize it." He explains that "we" always speed past this place on the expressway. "There's a wall about the southern tip of the Bronx.

It is not formed by the L tracks, or by the rivers, or the curve of the raised expressway that speeds us on its way. . . . It is a gray wall that whispers, 'Here: nothing.' But the wall itself is a lie." More long shots of the neighborhood follow, showing the train circuiting the city. "Within these five square miles, there's nothing—but 350,000 New Yorkers." The narrator's "we" addresses a white middle-class audience—those who believe in this myth of the wall.

The next shot frames a young man looking out the front train car onto the tracks: The film is now shooting from inside the train rather than observing it from outside, his gaze, perhaps, aligning with the camera's. Latin soul music emerges on the audio. The film intercuts rapidly back and forth between silent shots of residents looking out from their apartment windows and shots from inside the train accompanied by music. This intercutting ends on a scene of a young boy flying a kite from the rooftop, as a different man states, "I wish people could, uh, just tie me up like they do with a kite and fly me. . . . You know? Maybe that would solve a whole lot of problems. . . . I like it up there. I just cut the string, so they can't pull me back down." The narration has moved from an externalized observer of the area to the perspective of someone "on the inside," with the audio accompaniment of Latin music suggesting this someone is Puerto Rican. With these final intro segment words spoken by a Puerto Rican man, the narration has been handed off from outsider to insider.

The film's title then appears over this image of the kite. After this, we cut to scenes on the sidewalks. The narrator returns to explain that a neighborhood that "used to be primarily Jewish and Irish, with some others, is now primarily others." Different men speak about their experience of the changing neighborhood; their words are racist, shot through with references to African jungles, deterioration, undesirables. We are hearing the words, it is clear, of the older residents, presumably Jewish and Irish. One of them says, "How come they don't speak American?"; another man emphasizes the importance of "learning American." The narrator then states, "But thousands here speak American, and still the doors stay shut." The scene shifts to a market that is open to the street. Again, the audio moves among different speakers, as the visuals show women and children selecting among fruits and paying the vendor. Most of these speakers voice negative impressions of "Black people," for example, claiming that Black children steal groceries. The narrator again intercedes, saying that when welfare checks arrive, these people are targets for salesmen, who descend upon them, take their money, and go.

This is the last we hear from the implied older neighbors. Until the film's end, we hear the voices of Puerto Rican and Black residents, with only an intermittent voice-over from the narrator. Residents explain the tribulations of debilitated life—rats biting babies in their cribs, poor housing conditions—as well as the joys of their lives. For example, over visuals of men and boys playing stickball in the street, a resident says, "It's a good feeling. I know that.... You enjoy it! It's a sweet kick." The narrator then repeats, "It's a sweet kick, at 2 p.m. on a Wednesday afternoon, smack in the middle of the work-week. Who are these Wednesday ball players? The left fielder will be thirty-three next month. At midnight he may take the train downtown to his job, at a hash house." Later, scenes show residents, decked out in Saturday-night finery, window shopping; then, they attend a Federico García Lorca play. The narrator says that for those who do not live there the night appears as a danger-ous chaos, but for the residents, it's another night—there may be junkies, the narrator says, but they are just neighbors who are having a particularly hard time. Thus the narrator intervenes to say that white stereotypes are incorrect. The narrator's words—the use of "we"; his neutral inflection and unmarked accent—address a presumed middle-class, white viewer, one for whom the South Bronx is unknown, contained behind a wall. While the film includes voices of its documented subjects, they are re-objectified through this over-arching narratorial whiteness and the racial frame it evokes.

Understanding that this training material was created for incoming "in-digenous," nonprofessional workers—that is, people for whom there was no "wall"—suggests that the film's producers aimed to inculcate in trainees a habitus of middle-class professionalism. Peck and Struening's report indicates they were anxious over trainees' comportment and affective styles. After un-dergoing an initial battery of tests, applicants were "screened" for personality characteristics. In their summary of those tests, Peck and Struening conclude that their applicants exhibited different "cognitive styles" than those of the middle-class groups they had studied—to be specific, they concluded that the applicants "tend to use extreme categories of response."[9] The following section of this report summarizes the training program for these new em-ployees and includes mention of two films produced for Lincoln Hospital that these trainees watched. That *Uptown* oscillates between an insider's view of the South Bronx and an outsider's gaze at it resonates with the training pro-gram's implicit goal of transforming applicants with "extreme categories of re-sponse" into employees who would exhibit a white, middle-class professional demeanor. As they later state, the "concept of the indigenous worker," for Peck and Struening, "is still developing.... The role of the community mental health worker is ... [a] person who is in direct contact with both the commu-nity and the mental health professionals while in many ways remaining a peer of the client."[10] Peck and Struening hoped to capitalize on this bifurcation—

and learn from these new workers more about their community—but also feared it was detrimental to the functioning of their professional workplace. *Uptown* fit Peck and Struening's concepts of sufficient training media specifically because it cultivated a distanced, white gaze toward the Puerto Rican community. This gaze would inculcate a professional demeanor absent of the affective responses Peck and Struening deemed unprofessional.

The reviewer of the film for *Psychiatric Services* assessed the film's potential as a teaching tool. "The film serves as an introduction to this subculture for persons who may be training to work in mental health services in similarly deprived areas. If the film implies that a large number of these people may need psychiatric help, it also shows that there are others who may be potential indigenous nonprofessional workers."[11] The film-critical gaze wielded by the discipline itself thus employed a psychiatric way of screening that distinguished between those who were designated pathological and those who could enter the profession.

Feminist-of-Color Information Justice

The feminist-of-color activism for information justice at Lincoln Hospital did not take the same form such activism takes in our current moment, for example, in activist efforts against algorithmic injustice or around predictive artificial intelligence (AI). Nor were the efforts that I here synthesize as information justice activism articulated by feminist-of-color activists through that concept, either at the time or in their later histories of the events. In naming these efforts "information activism," this section argues that feminist-of-color organizing included an implicit challenge to information injustice. The argument therefore adds to two strands of intellectual work: first, emerging studies that destabilize the centrality of white men to histories of computing, and that foreground the role of the mundane labor of information in social justice movements; second, feminist genealogies of technology and information.[12]

The nonprofessional workers at Lincoln Hospital Mental Health Services objected to the information system that governed their daily work. Lincoln Hospital's information system was a biopolitical, racial-pathologizing project, evident in contemporaneous reports about the system and in research later published from data that the system gathered. In that same report to NIMH in which Peck and Struening summarized how they tested job applicants, they reported on their endeavors to incorporate computers into their research practices. This computerization of community mental health centers was by no means singular to Lincoln Hospital; it was, in fact, a central part of New York State's plans to modernize mental health facilities. The Health and Mental Hygiene Facilities Improvement Corporation, appointed by the New York governor to spend $700 million that the New York legislature approved for designing and building hospitals and health centers, reported on their guiding principles for all New York State mental health facilities. The report's section that explicitly addressed computers was accompanied by images of Lincoln Hospital's planned new facilities. Its author first noted how increased construction costs and new technological advances "press rapidly upon one another." Then, "Often . . . modern[izing] facilities . . . makes possible a more efficient structuring of health care delivery systems. [Innovations in design include] automation to improve the quality of medical care and lower the cost of providing it, including computers that operate patient care information systems as an aid in diagnosis, perform chemical analysis in laboratories, keep records, schedule staffs and plan menus."[13] For the state administrators tasked with spending state funding to address outdated and dilapidated mental health services facilities, computerization was embedded into their imaginary of modernization and revitalization.

This same report noted that the architectural firm of Max O. Urbahn (also a consultant on *Bold New Approach*, discussed in chapter 1) had been contracted to draw up architectural plans for a new Lincoln Medical Center, one of six "health projects" the corporation was designing, with automation a central feature of the center's planning. That new hospital would not see fruition in the immediately following years, even though it was well known among both city administrators and the local community that Lincoln Hospital was in decrepit shape—its filth, lead-painted walls, overcrowding, and general deteriorated status were decried during the many activist challenges from 1969 through 1971. There was certainly overall agreement, by both city administrators and community members, that Lincoln Hospital needed to be rebuilt; for some staff and community members, the delay in moving forward with the rebuilding signaled the city's dedication to the health empire, rather than the health of the people. Of interest to me here is that city administrators envisioned a new building organized around computers, yet this was not the kind of remodel that workers, doctors, or patients wanted. Lincoln Hospital had last undergone a major remodel in 1934, and its electrical system dated from the 1920s, meaning power consistently went out.[14] Surgical rooms often had no air-conditioning. Electrical updates, not computers, were the urgent need. In the early 1960s, administrators removed waiting-room seating to install ten microfilm machines, for the stated purpose of managing patient records. Yet there was neither room for the machines nor staff who knew how to use them. As Fitzhugh Mullan, an LHMHS psychiatrist, describes this event in his memoir, management had made a decision about technology without consulting staff, a harbinger of more to come.[15]

In 1963, when program planners at Albert Einstein affiliated with Lincoln Hospital, they included among their five services "a research department," as well as "a system that would reveal when and where a client enters the service network and what happens to him; that would lend itself to measurement of program reach, efficiency and effectiveness."[16] There was no model in existence on which to build, and so, when the OEO funded the neighborhood service centers, they applied to NIMH for and were granted funding to develop a record system. After more than six months creating, assessing, and revising coding and forms, in 1966 LHMHS administrators rolled out their computer program, which ran on IBM computers. When administrators first instituted their recordkeeping system at the neighborhood service centers, staff resisted; as the administrators put it, "There was some initial resistance to data collection among the NSC [Neighborhood Service Center] staff, particularly the non-professionals who were so highly motivated to give direct help to community residents that they were not at first able to see a relationship between data-collection they conceived to be time-consuming and the ultimate efficiency to their function."[17] Nevertheless, workers had no choice but to comply. "Involvement of . . . workers in the actual development of the record system . . . was not merely a strategy to commit them but was essential since we were . . . dependent upon them for descriptions of their procedures and assessments of forms as they were piloted. . . . A research staff member was almost continuously on hand at the NSC for consultation and interpretation of what we needed from them and how we would use the data."[18] Dedicated staff were hired to oversee programming and to transfer data from written forms to punch cards.[19]

By 1968, the computer system was fully supporting the LHMHS's research program, which was staffed by an anthropologist, a demographer, social psychologists, and research assistants, as well as part-time staff and many graduate student researchers. Peck and Struening's 1968 report summarized the process as follows: "The record system receives constant monitoring. Before cards are punched, the forms are examined and errors corrected and omissions supplied. Although the forms appear complex, the community mental health workers consider them fairly simple to complete; the exactness of the explanations and the definition of each point have contributed to this. General training sessions are held whenever changes are made in procedures or when clarification is needed."[20] In a 1968 assessment of research in community psychiatry, Jerome Collins, MD, of the Biomedical Stress Research Branch of the US Army Medical Research and Development Command, reported on a recent visit to Lincoln:

> The most important element of the Lincoln Hospital Project is the collection of accurate data at the Neighborhood Service Centers. Data are collected on a series of carefully designed forms that the *indigenous nonprofessional workers complete*—an initial-contact form, a service-rendered form, a staff-activity form, and a narrative form. All the forms can be easily and quickly completed.... Clinicians and administrators at all levels have to cooperate actively to ensure that the data collected are accurate and complete.... [W]hen I visited the research staff..., they confessed that there were still many technological problems to be solved. (Emphasis added)[21]

Also in 1968 a new IBM computer, the IBM 360, arrived, and research staff modified their in-house software for it.[22]

These reports' self-applause masks how the computerized system and the data-recording requirements it created exacerbated workplace tensions. At both Lincoln Hospital and LHMHS, the occupational hierarchy was stratified by race, gender, and class. The well-paid white administrators oversaw grossly underpaid nonprofessional workers who were mostly Puerto Rican and Black. In other words, computers aggravated ongoing tensions between Albert Einstein as a place of white middle-class experts who viewed Lincoln Hospital as a research opportunity and LHMHS as a place of working-class-of-color staff who viewed their work as an opportunity for care. A glance through the codebook and forms provided to community mental health workers reveals the burdensome nature of the paperwork: In addition to the usual notes in narrative form, every contact with a client required filling out more than twenty pages of forms and using numerical codes drawn from a fifty-four page codebook.[23] The data being recorded were more oriented toward research into demographics and incidence rates—public and population health issues—than patient care. And nonprofessional workers also had to document, over seven pages, the allocation of their own work time for each week. To staff, these additional seven pages indicated that their own labor was being fed into the data regime. Staff were certainly aware that they were research subjects for their supervisors, part of the Great Society experiment in whether Puerto Rican and Black community members could be trained to enact the biopolitics of Great Society ideologies.

It is also highly probable that staff were fully aware of the racializing and pathologizing logics embedded within the research Peck and Struening were conducting. An example research article that grew from this research is their "Migration and Ethnic Membership in Relation to Social Problems," published in *American Behavioral Scientist*. The article analyzed data on mental health admissions in the Bronx and Brooklyn, as well as health-related data such as infant deaths and "deviant behavior," to enter an ongoing discussion over "the relationship between migration and mental illness." The authors hoped to produce knowledge that would allow "the ability to predict the future distribution of social problems among the sectors of our great cities[, which] would seem to be of obvious importance if we are to adequately plan and subsequently evaluate programs of intervention and reconstruction."[24] (Bizarrely, in their analysis of higher rates of hospitalization from 1961 to 1965, the authors failed to note that there had also been an increase in mental health services, which in and of itself might explain the greater rates of hospitalization.)

For three days in 1969, the first of many direct-action events occurred. Mental health workers, janitorial staff, and administrators of color took over the mental health clinic. Published summaries of this event named the recordkeeping system as an instigating factor. The influential *American Health Empire* (1970) argued that workers viewed data extraction as subtracting from time that was better spent caring for their clients, and a 1973 book argued that the nonprofessional workers thought data were being used to surveil their job performance.[25] Both of these probably contributed to the actions. Perhaps aggravating the situation too was the surveillance of workers that began even before they were hired—when applicants interviewed for the nonprofessional worker positions, professionals observed and assessed them through a one-way mirror.[26] In May 1970, worker-activists mounted a counterveillance program: They established a twenty-four-hour complaints desk, staffed by Cleo Silvers and supported by workers who would follow patients from the desk into clinical areas of the hospital to document their complaints. In effect, the complaints desk gathered a new kind of database, one that counteracted administrators' surveillance of patients and workers with patients' and workers' counterveillance of hospital administrators.

The initial three-day 1969 action hastened a burgeoning feminist-of-color praxis and organizing among LHMHS workers. Across four New York City hospitals and health centers, workers of color formed the Health Revolutionary Unity Movement (HRUM). Co-led by Cleo Silvers, HRUM distanced itself from the local union, which would not support organizing on the ground at hospitals. Many HRUM members were also members of, or worked closely with, the Young Lords. In May 1970, members of the Young Lords and Lincoln Hospital members of HRUM formed the Think Lincoln Collective, which had as one primary goal challenging the Health and Hospital Corporation and its intention to consolidate, defund, and decrease staffing at Lincoln. While circulating information to patients and workers about these intentions, Silvers led the group to establish a complaints desk.

As the complaints desk gathered its data, on July 13, 1970, the Young Lords decided to take direct action and occupy the hospital. Although the Young Lords initiated the action, after they had control of the hospital, HRUM workers and the new residents, including a group of four progressive white residents who called themselves the Lincoln Collective, supported the action. Concluded after only twelve hours, nevertheless the takeover, where activists unfurled banners saying "Bienvenidos al hospital del pueblo" and "Welcome to the People's Hospital" and immediately instituted community screening for tuberculosis and lead poisoning, demonstrated the power of community demands for community control of care.

Less than a week later, activists would stage a new intervention into hospital information systems. This intervention became an urgent necessity after a patient died from medical negligence on July 17. During a clinical exam, Carmen Rodriguez, a woman well known to staff from her visits to its drug rehab clinic, was discovered to be pregnant; due to her rheumatic heart disease, which made pregnancy life-threatening, doctors scheduled her for an abortion at a later date. The new resident on call administered a saline solution abortion, well documented as a dangerous decision for patients with rheumatic heart disease. When Rodriguez began having breathing problems, the intern treated her for asthma with medicine that worsens heart disease issues. As Johanna Fernández's careful research into this event shows, Rodriguez was conscious and certainly knew she didn't have asthma; yet the resident, well trained in medical misogynoir, never consulted with her about either her treatment or her responses to it and continued with this ultimately lethal course of action.[27]

After Rodriguez's death, a psychiatrist (also a member of HRUM) reviewed her confidential record and, understanding the magnitude of negligence, shared it with the Think Lincoln Collective. Outraged, they demanded changes to hospital practices and a change of administrators.[28] The Young Lords then forced a remarkable event: A clinical pathological conference on Rodriguez's treatment was made public to community members, who packed the room to interrogate the multiple physicians debating her care. As one of the doctors present recounts the event, "It was a troubled, even tortured example of community control of medical services.... [It was] a victory for community participation in the hospital."²⁹ No doubt tortured because of the murder that inspired it, and troubling to a hospital empire that sought to obscure its abandonment, this People's Clinical Pathological Conference has been consistently noted as the first such event. It was remarkable in the people's refusal to allow the health empire its control over both information and its interpretation.

After Rodriguez's murder, the free newsletter of HRUM, *For the People's Health*, reported on Lincoln Hospital's ob/gyn services through the language of reproductive justice for Puerto Rican and Black women, and nationalist rhetorics of genocide. Certainly reproductive justice was already a developing framework of these feminists of color, and Rodriguez's murder, occurring during a time when their critiques of sexism within left activism were already affecting the Young Lords and the Lincoln Collective, heightened the urgency and relevance of their critique. What I want to emphasize here is HRUM's heightened and explicit demands, after Rodriguez's death, for continuity of care—that is, assigning one doctor to each patient, instead of the model that was in place in which a patient might be seen by multiple different people over the course of a stay or an illness. This was not their only demand, far from it. I wish to emphasize this because it appears that the (mostly white, mostly professional) Lincoln Collective joined the demand for continuity of care to a reformist aim of changing the hospital's recordkeeping system.

I say "appears" because the archival records contain some fuzziness around specific dates, likely due both to those records containing post hoc summaries as well as to the speed with which various crises at the hospital emerged. Nevertheless, the Lincoln Collective's summary of their July 1970 philosophy included collective decision-making, breaking down medical hierarchies (e.g., involving aides and nurses in decisions), and instituting continuity of care. That continuity of care would be supported through team rounds and a new medical recordkeeping system, the "Weed system."³⁰ First proposed in 1969 and now in widespread use, Lawrence Weed's Patient-Oriented Medical Record (POMR) tracked a patient's problems, treatment plan, and progress; it substituted for the conventional medical recordkeeping practice of tracking what tests had been ordered for a patient. As Weed proposed it, the POMR would allow for continuity of care and for input from more staff than only attending physicians. The appeal of the POMR for the Lincoln Collective is clear. Within Lincoln Hospital's highly stratified, hierarchical professional setting, the POMR increased the power of nurses and nonprofessional workers to contribute important information, including information that physicians, residents, and interns might ignore, to patient care. As the Lincoln Collective put it in an undated newsletter, "On each chart the first problem is always well child care, and we make every effort to begin to deal with those parts of the diseases of oppression usually defined as outside the conventional medical sphere."[31] Whether borne directly out of feminist-of-color demands that reproductive justice required continuity of care or not, nevertheless, the new left group of Lincoln Collective articulated a change to the health empire's information system in relation to a politics of care and information.

Even so, this reformist information system did not solve broader infrastructural issues. A few months later, the pediatrics unit of the Lincoln Collective criticized what they saw as poor use of the Weed system. They connected this poor use to a lack of both teaching and mentoring relationships, as well as a general laziness about patient well-being. "This attitude [of laziness] leads to... [f]ailure of the house staff member in many instances to have his mind challenged in considering a difficult diagnostic problem by someone who can many times provide him with additional information and stimuli. Also they lead to inadequate recordkeeping with many of us only using the Weed System in a primitive automated fashion. This causes a narrowing of our understanding of the patients' problems."[32] A change to information systems perceived as radical could not institute radical changes without broader structural changes.

Another development from these events was the eventual replacement of the authoritative administrator by Dr. Helen Rodriguez-Trías. A pediatrician trained in Puerto Rico and exposed to the rampant sterilization of Puerto Rican women there, Rodriguez-Trías would, within a few years after joining Lincoln Hospital, found the Committee to End Sterilization Abuse. In reports about her early years at Lincoln Hospital, Rodriguez-Trías wrote of the Health and Hospitals Corporation's move to computerized forms and billing with polite disdain: "These, I am afraid, are not as efficient as they should be, but it has basically not improved the quality of care."[33]

The information justice activism at Lincoln Hospital was, at each turn, supported by the feminist-of-color critique of Lincoln Hospital and other hospitals in this health empire, a critique that was developing among Young Lords members and HRUM members. Documented in Morales's *Through the Eyes of Rebel Women* and in Fitzhugh Mullan's memoir, feminist-of-color critique affected both the Young Lords and the Lincoln Collective, who worked to integrate its critique of patriarchal hierarchies within radical collectives. Feminist-of-color critique of the health empire was also articulated in *For the People's Health*. The free newsletter regularly reported on disparities in pay

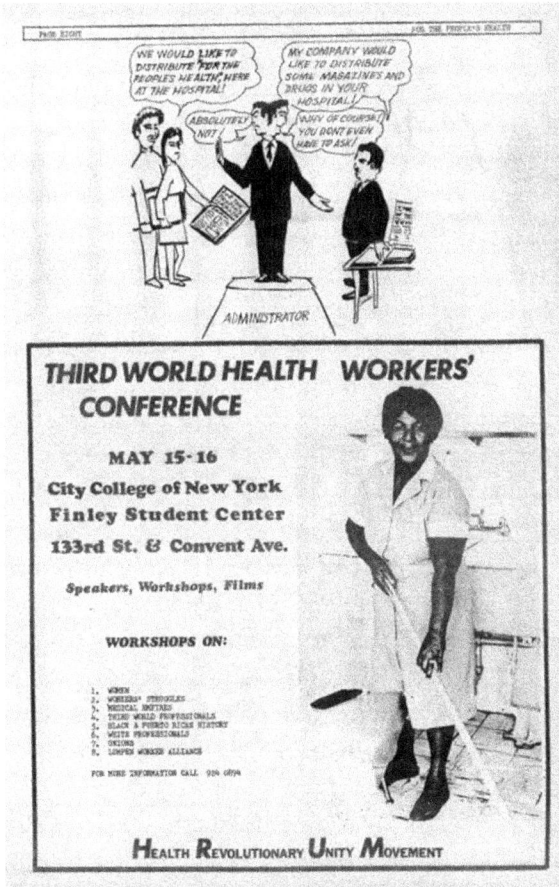

FIGURE 2.1. *For the People's Health* (March 9, 1971).

and on racialized and gendered hierarchies of occupational positions. A cartoon from a 1971 issue slyly encodes a feminist-of-color feminist critique of how information figured into the hospital-as-empire (fig. 2.1). At the center of the cartoon appears a man in a suit, standing on a platform that says "Administrator"; hydra-headed, the man speaks on his right to a company representative, also dressed in a suit, and on the left his other head addresses a man and a woman, the duo possibly dressed in nurse uniforms. To the right, the company representative asks permission to distribute magazines and drugs, which the administrator enthusiastically grants; to the left, the woman asks for permission to distribute *For the People's Health*, which the administrator decisively refuses. In other words, in order to maintain its health empire the hospital retains tight control over how and what information flows within it.[34] That a woman makes the demand of the administrator to distribute *For the People's Health* is suggestive of how a woman-of-color stance challenges the health empire's information systems. This cartoon appears above an announcement of the upcoming Third World Health Workers' Conference. That announcement includes a list of workshops, with "Women" its top entry, and an image of a uniformed woman of color mopping a bathroom floor. The juxtaposition of these two genres—the cartoon and the informational announcement—cannily highlights the function of the newsletter itself as a radical information system. The hospital refuses the newsletter's distribution in order to suppress feminist-of-color organizing.

Finally, an additional demand advanced by HRUM was the Patient's Bill of Rights, which has become ubiquitous on US hospital-room walls after the American Hospital Association's 1974 adoption of (a watered-down version of) it. HRUM's Patient's Bill of Rights was the first successful articulation of patients as citizens with rights that include patient dignity, medically ethical treatment, and transparency in care.[35] That a group led by feminists of color first advanced these rights, taken for granted by many today, is a significant (if now often-unacknowledged) history. Among the ten rights enumerated is the right "to have access to your medical chart." In this right, we can locate another instance of information activism: a demand for the right to information that the hospital traditionally controlled.

In the many accounts of these years of activism at Lincoln Hospital, when feminist-of-color critique has been centered, it has not been articulated to information activism. Yet that critique and the women building it had profound influence, in ways both direct and indirect, on every new intervention into the health empire's biopolitics of information. Silvers staffed the counterveillant complaint table; female HRUM workers connected their struggles to change workplace hierarchies to the politics of reproductive justice, which then affected how radicalized white professionals thought about information systems; HRUM workers understood their newsletter as a form of information activism that could disrupt the health empire's information systems; their ongoing struggle for community control, guided by feminist practices and principles, succeeding in ousting several administrators; they appointed a Puerto Rican leader who would lead the charge in reproductive justice politics throughout the 1970s; they demanded that medical information be open to patients themselves; and HRUM's challenges to the white male physicians of the Lincoln Collective, which its members expressed by insisting the Lincoln Collective join in the struggle to challenge gendered wage disparities, shifted the collective toward a more radical organizing stance and toward implementing workplace practices in which education and care practices were more equally distributed.

Feminist-of-color organizing also transformed mediated representations of Puerto Rican health, as well as the filmmaking practices of a radical filmmaking collective.

Newsreel's *Lincoln Hospital*: Montage Against Binary

As both Johanna Fernández and Cynthia Young have shown, the Young Lords understood the power of the image and of the mass media.[36] The Lords often tipped off New York journalists to upcoming actions, securing themselves news coverage. They also invited members of the radical filmmaking collective Newsreel to accompany them when they occupied the Methodist Church; footage from this event appears in the Newsreel film *El pueblo se levanta* (1971). Newsreel members were also present during the worker struggle at Lincoln Hospital in 1969. That footage was included in the 1971 film *Lincoln Hospital*. Although the films of Newsreel, and of its successor collective, Third World Newsreel, are well documented and theorized in film studies and American studies, *Lincoln Hospital* remains little discussed.[37] But, for multiple reasons, the film deserves careful attention. First, it intervened in mainstream representations of Puerto Ricans and in mainstream reporting on the Lincoln Hospital struggles, and thus, as insurgent media, it extends our understandings of radical filmmaking of the time. Second, made during Newsreel's transformation from a white-centered, new left collective to a third-world collective, the film deserves consideration for its role in that transformation—including how the events they filmed may have crystallized for Newsreel members that radical US health politics connected to third-world health politics. Third, *Lincoln Hospital* joins with *El pueblo se levanta* and *Rompiendo puertas* (1970), a Newsreel film about a women-of-color–led occupation of New York housing, to articulate left politics with third-world politics, and, in a move new to Newsreel productions, to formally articulate it through the heightened presence of a woman narrator.

The film's opening montage, which cuts between title cards and exterior scenes of the South Bronx, stages a more direct confrontation with the data of health abandonment than *Uptown* does. The eleven-minute film opens to white text on a black screen that reads "THE SOUTH BRONX / 30% black, 70% Puerto Rican / WESTCHESTER COUNTY / 98% White." Two exterior shots of storefronts follow; pedestrians, dressed in overcoats, pass on the sidewalk.

More titles: "The average income of THE SOUTH BRONX is half that of WEST-CHESTER COUNTY"; "The infant mortality rate of THE SOUTH BRONX is double that of WESTCHESTER COUNTY"; "WESTCHESTER COUNTY has 1 hospital bed per 93 people; THE SOUTH BRONX has 1 hospital bed per 4,500 people"; "WESTCHESTER COUNTY has 28 private, and 1 public hospital. THE SOUTH BRONX has no private, and 1 public hospital: Lincoln Hospital." These frames intersect with shots of the storefronts. Throughout, Puerto Rican music plays, with distinctly martial drumbeats.

Like *Uptown*, the film begins with statistics that emphasize the stark contrast between different areas of New York. Unlike *Uptown*'s comparison of multiple different areas of New York, *Lincoln Hospital* contrasts solely a wealth-privileged white area to the impoverished area of color. The use of both lowercased words and capitalization for the two areas is akin to a computer's binary logic, and its visual distinction between a category of uppercase and one of lowercase mimics a tab-stopped entry form. This dualistic contrast foregrounds how wealth and ethnicity determine health. It is also suggestive of binary logic: the data-driven discourse and statistical project that underwrote Lincoln Hospital's research agenda, and state biopolitics more broadly. In referencing statistics, these opening title frames echo the logic of the gaze of the clinic—where the physician, or psychiatrist, focuses on the patient as a series of charts, data, and test results rather than as a human being. As I explore here, the film's conclusion unwinds this binary logic and clinical gaze, offering, through collective images, a proliferation of meaning that escapes its technological capture.

After these intercut sequences, over a broad exterior shot of Lincoln Hospital that pans from its foundations to its top floors, two narrators are heard. The voices of a male and a female narrator explain the affiliation plan and what they call "Lincoln Hospital's mental health services *experiment*," which includes the training of paraprofessionals—then rephrased, with emphasis, as *non*professionals—to work at the mental health services' storefronts. This information is delivered with shots of the one-way mirror interviewee assessment setting, a visual that, by depicting their surveillance by professional workers, underscores the demotion implied by the term "nonprofessional." Throughout, both narrators use the first-person plural—"we"—to indicate they are the nonprofessionals. The film therefore articulates itself as conveying the voice of Puerto Rican workers at Lincoln Hospital.

They succinctly deliver a radical critique of the health empire: "The politicians decided that they couldn't manage the city hospitals, so in 1961, the city government thought up something called the affiliation plan. Seven private medical schools and centers took over the management of twenty public hospitals." The next words are uttered by a female narrator in voice-over. "Their argument was that the private medical schools were more efficient, but really, their plan made the hospitals even less responsible to the communities they were supposed to serve." The next shot returns to the same exterior street location, this time panning to observe a young woman using crutches. Another title appears: "Under the AFFILIATION PLAN: Albert Einstein School of Medicine Manages Lincoln Hospital." The male voice narrates as the visuals cut to a man in a white lab coat walking past a bust of Einstein: "Hospitals like Lincoln Hospital have always been slaughterhouses, but now they're slaughterhouses run by medical schools." The narrator continues: Because Einstein considers itself a progressive institution, it has "a whole number of programs designed to, quote, involve the community." After describing the comprehensive mental health services provided in these programs, another male narrator explains, "They trained us as part of this new program, new careers for the poor. We were a new job category, paraprofessionals." "The program got one million dollars from the Office of Economic Opportunity," he says. The female narrator returns: "But it became clear that most of the programs were paper, designed to pull in private and federal grants." Him: "Albert Einstein used us." Her: "We were just window-dressing for Albert Einstein's liberal reputation." An alarm sounds, the screen fades to black, and the words THE NEWSREEL blink on-screen several times to the martial sound of bullets (Newsreel's signature credit sequence). The alarm returns, and the scene opens on a gathering of police vans parked near protestors, marching in front of Lincoln Hospital.

The film's visuals of South Bronx sidewalks, its extra-diegetic music, and its first-person plural narration by Lincoln Hospital workers establish that the film emanates from the people. In this, the film clearly rejects, from the outset, documentaries about urban life that are authorized by white narrators. Additionally, with the martial sound of bullets in Newsreel's signature title sequence as well as the sound of an alarm (possibly of an ambulance), the film also rejects an aesthetic based in sympathy, sentiment, or positive affects—the register of racial liberalism. Instead, *Lincoln Hospital*'s aesthetics announce its intent to rupture and challenge.

The rest of the film documents the Lincoln Hospital takeover. Scenes show an organizer handing out paper and a table at which people sit filling out forms. Over this, a male narrator explains, "It's like people taking over a factory and producing. They're actually giving something to the community and showing that there's a new way to handle a strike. A strike doesn't have to be just walking out on the services." Throughout, their actions are described as community control of services, control that was asserted after four years of frustrations with the hospital, "four years where we tried to do real work, in a paper program." Another female voice explains that their children's services office has a huge waitlist: When children come in, they fill out forms, then send them to other clinics. Other problems detailed are the daytime hours for therapy, which do not align with neighborhood residents' work schedules; and the lack of funding for taxi fares, making it time-prohibitive to visit people at their homes, a requirement of good care work. The next sequence includes the voices of clients. A woman asks, in a heated voice, why people do not improve over two years of return visits but instead are walking around "like zombies, full of dope, and I'm talking about medicine." The next sequence shows a client's apartment. Children play on a tiled floor as the male narrator explains that in their work they would often help people with rat-infested apartments, moving them if necessary—until "word came down from The Man to cool it. We found out later the landlord contributed to Albert Einstein." Then, with the male and female narrators rotating, they describe how, even if they could run the facility, and at night, they still wouldn't have enough money to do what needed to be done, "because we're talking about a whole system that conspires to keep people sick." The alarm sounds again, and the film cuts to the protests and takeover, with diegetic sound as an administrator, surrounded by protestors, attempts to respond to their demands. A narrator returns. "We don't want to run more efficient, bad health care. We're talking about a different definition of health. Health isn't anything mysterious. It isn't a drug company's financial reports, or research on the masses. It's strong bodies, good minds, and people being treated as people." Flamenco music accompanies a series of still images of the faces of community members, and the film ends on a still image of a man at a podium, arm raised aloft, holding a piece of paper: a list of demands.

The film's formal elements, like many other Newsreel films of this time, draw from third-world cinema: jump cuts; direct address; a sonic motif of militancy; cinéma verité. They also join characteristics of the white new left (radical, antiwar folk music) with those of the third world (Puerto Rican music), thus sonically evincing what Cynthia Young argues was a growing shift in Newsreel's film practice of articulating new left to third-world concerns.[38] Unlike Newsreel's *Finally Got the News*, where the voices of Black women are contained to one segment, *Lincoln Hospital* mixes male and female voices throughout the narration. Its filmmakers had clearly learned, from criticism made by women members of the collective that *Finally Got the News* had consigned women's voices to a short, separate segment, that its voice-representational choices were a form of gender politics.[39] With narration provided by multiple participants in the workers' struggle, the film's narration constitutes a multivocal and multigendered public.

The visuals also support the narration's clear message: Structural racism—inherent to urban real estate, medical institutions, Big Pharma, and paltry urban funding for life-sustaining services—is better named as infrastructural, institutional racism, in which each social institution feeds the other's systems for maintaining oppression. This is vitally clear when the film's narration highlights that the connections between the real estate industry and the hospital and medical school industries prohibit caring for the health of community members, over visuals showing the interior of a run-down apartment where children play on its filthy floor. It is also emphasized in the many shots that emphasize the monumentality of those industries' built environment: its introductory exterior shot of a massive hospital building; shots of Albert Einstein's surrounding concrete-paved outdoor areas, which are wide open spaces in which a lone white-coated doctor looks diminutive. These shots convey the enormous material space occupied by these industries, their brutal heft that demotes humans and promotes industry. The film's concluding series of still images of human faces emphasizes that its radical health activist critique of structures, institutions, and systems promotes a collectivity of humans, where individual members achieve health when the health of all is supported.

Additionally, two key moments in the film's narrative arc—its introduction, with a sequence of still frames filled with text; and its conclusion, a series of freeze-frames of faces that climaxes with a single figure in a pose of militancy holding aloft a piece of paper with a list of demands—are aesthetic choices that move from binary and clinical logic to communitarian logic. The opening uses a rhetoric of statistics within a dualistic logic, emphasizing the binary logic of the computer that underlies medical research, and its dependence on numbers for knowledge mirrors the clinical gaze that underpins research. In contrast, the closing series stitches together a multiplicity of human faces, a community that has emerged, through the work of struggle, from the limited-origin point of data rhetoric into the unlimited, public collective space of demand. Although the film does not explicitly name HRUM's struggle around computers and recordkeeping, a struggle for a filmic mode of representation that contests the clinic's *research logics* informs this final sequence. This is why the final series is shorn of guiding narration or discursive-linguistic explanatory frames. Rather than circle back to the film's introductory numerical and linguistic mode of representation, this final sequence insists on a cinematic language, which refutes the computer's—and the clinic's—logic of correspondence. That is, where the computer and the clinic view signs as corresponding to the signified—viewing data as indicative of one meaning, in a one-to-one correspondence of sign to meaning—the collective series of images proliferates meaning, suturing and cleaving, opening new possibilities.

There is an argument to be made that these formal choices were determined by radical aesthetics that eschewed all adornment and metaphor as bourgeois. Even if my earlier reading has pressed the film to an interpretation it was not meant to bear, its allusion to and revision of the opening statistical sequence of Danska's *Uptown* are nonetheless meaningful. The film creates a stark contrast between care in two racialized populations and the political-geographic area where they live, and, in doing so, *Lincoln Hospital* frames *the hospital's educational cinema* (recall that *Uptown* was produced for Lincoln) as participating in, rather than rupturing, the pathologizing capacity of the health empire's media and technologies. Yet if exposing how pedagogical medical media racialized and debilitated required the polar oppositional logic that could reify the binary as a mode of articulation, the film's concluding sequence challenges this logic: The struggle for community control documented in the body of the film produces a logic of collectivity, represented through a uniquely cinematic language. Community control redirects clinical attention to caring for people, rather than taking care of data.

Little has been written about *Lincoln Hospital*, either in histories of health and media activism or in film studies scholarship on Newsreel. The two other Newsreel films about Puerto Rican activism produced at this same time, *El pueblo se levanta* and *Rompiendo puertas*, have received little attention as well. Their most thoughtful analysis appears in Young's *Soul Power: Culture, Radicalism, and the Making of a US Third World Left*, where Young contextualizes them within scholarship on the relationship between the new left, working-class movements, and the rise of a third-world left. For Young, these two films in particular serve to complicate traditional film historical work on Newsreel, because they demonstrate that in 1969–72 Newsreel began to shift from its hierarchical, white male leadership model of production to one where its female members and members of color held more sway; because of this, the films it collectively decided to produce covered issues within working-class communities of color. For example, while the well-known Newsreel production *Columbia Revolt* (1968) centers white college students as the chief actors, thus buttressing vanguard theories of radical struggle, the aesthetics and formal elements of the later *El pueblo se levanta* and *Rompiendo puertas* center a community struggle arising from multiple actors, depicting radical struggle as multivocal, multiethnic, and led as much by women as by men.

El pueblo se levanta and *Rompiendo puertas* would, as Young argues, mark a significant turn in Newsreel's own practice from a white-led filmmaking collective to one led by filmmakers of color who articulated US radical politics to a third-world, anticolonial movement, and articulated a third-world critique through a feminist-of-color perspective—a perspective that developed, by 1979, into a film discussed in chapter 4 that explicitly articulated feminist-of-color critique to third-world feminism. In recovering *Lincoln Hospital*, this chapter argues that it was not only their work with the Young Lords for *El pueblo se levanta* that occasioned this shift; it was also prompted by Newsreel's work with women-of-color workers at the hospital, who were developing a resolute critique of the health empire's classed, racialized, and gender politics. The importance of the film as a form of insurgent media meant to circulate and educate struggles elsewhere is indicated in the fact that, when Newsreel transformed to Third World Newsreel, *Lincoln Hospital* remained in its catalog.

The sites of struggle over media and technology at Lincoln Hospital that this chapter excavates reveal that activism for community control of health and its mediations pervaded *all* media-technological domains at Lincoln Hospital, not only the more commonly expected domain of film. Most importantly, these struggles arose from feminist-of-color critique, which either directly intervened in these sites or implicitly reshaped the politics of all activists involved, including the Young Lords and the Lincoln Collective. This chapter thus joins with other work that rethinks histories of information systems and their attendant media. From their newsletters, to their complaint desks, to their People's Clinical Pathological Conference, feminists of color organized against a racial pathologizing politics of information. They articulated health information systems and health media as infrastructures of domination and pathologization.

3

FROM SPILLOVER TO STREETS

Community-Organized Filmmaking as Mutual Aid

For eight weeks in 1970, an integrated film crew shot *Hitch: Portrait of a Black Leader as a Young Man* on location in Harlem. The film, produced and directed by mental health film director Irving Jacoby and cowritten with Black Arts intellectual and artist Julian Mayfield, was made to promote the Northside Center for Child Development, a mental health services center in Harlem run by Black psychologists Kenneth and Mamie Clark. During those eight weeks, two Northside Center volunteers and local community organizers, Sam Gaynor and Sam Walton, accompanied the shoot, observing the media-making process. In the following years, Gaynor and Walton would use their newly acquired filmmaking knowledge to write, produce, and direct *Sam, Sam and Harlem* (1974), a documentary about their own Black self-help organization, We Care. These two films had limited circulation and almost no contemporaneous press coverage; although one is mentioned in Gerald Markowitz and David Rosner's exhaustive history of the Northside Center, they have not been discussed in American studies, film historical studies, or disability studies. Recovering these two films, this chapter unearths how Black cultural production intervened in the politics of "mental health/illness" and discourses of "Black pathologies" during this era. These films advanced a Black disability politics of "mental health" care. In the case of Gaynor and Walton's documentary, the film articulated such a politics to Black self-determination of media. And they connected a Black media politics to information activism.

The recovery of these films thus expands two strands of emergent disability studies scholarship. First, these films clarify what Sami Schalk names as an emergent "Black disability politics" of this era, that is, "anti-ableist arguments and actions performed by black cultural workers which address disability within the contexts of anti-black racism."[1] Schalk argues that Black activists did not express these disability politics through concepts coming to the fore in (white-centered) disability (and gay) activism (identity, pride, etc.). Indeed, the films discussed here shied away from such language entirely. In fact, even as they countered psychiatric discourse and narratives, they eschewed the rhetoric and concepts of antipsychiatry, of the emerging psychiatric survivor groups, and of alternative therapeutic movements. This elision underscores that a Black disability politics focused on "mental health" had a different genealogy from these other, white-oriented movements. The Black disability politics of mental health that these films advance constitute an incipient crip-of-color critique, to draw from Jina B. Kim.[2] Being designated "mentally ill," "mad," or otherwise deviant was not an identity to reclaim. Rather, the films represented how intersections of racism, sanism, and ableism pathologized Black life and supported policies that denied life-giving resources to Black communities. These independent media-makers challenged the reigning discourse of Black pathology that derived from histories of medical and psychiatric racism and from social scientific discourses of the "tangle of pathology."

Second, these films add to recent discussions about cripping film and media studies and about race and nontheatrical cinema.[3] These two feature-length films implicitly responded to and countered the narratives about Black communities in state-sponsored educational films, which reproduced tropes and discourses about Blackness as pathological and gave added fuel to policies that deprived impoverished communities of color of resources. Producing countervisions to such state-sponsored films was an urgent matter. These films thus add a new valence to discussions of disability and cinema. They demonstrate that the history of disability and cinema is not as white as it might seem—that in fact Black media-makers, even with the extraordinary challenges of becoming trained and employed in the media industries, developed representational and narrative strategies to articulate a Black disability politics.[4]

I begin with a brief analysis of one state-produced pedagogical film, *A Day in the Death of Donny B.* (dir. Carl Fick; 1969). Then, I undertake a comparative analysis of *Hitch* and *Sam, Sam and Harlem*. A film with competing narrative and ideological dynamics, *Hitch* demonstrates the pressure on independent media-makers to conform to tropes and motifs that would satisfy audiences of different political commitments, including potential donors. *Sam, Sam and Harlem* develops what I call a vernacular aesthetics of mutual aid. The documentary's aesthetics, rooted in the everyday and quotidian, refused the visual, rhetorical, and narrative logics of mental health cinema. Reading *Hitch* and *Sam, Sam and Harlem* across their different visions of Harlem and in regard to their complicated production histories, this chapter reveals the industrial and aesthetic pressures negotiated by Black media-makers who sought to produce countervisions of mental distress and its care.

Mental Hygiene Cinema as State Promotional Film

This section briefly outlines the racializing project of state-funded mental hygiene cinema. In the post–World War II era, mental hygiene film productions soared in number. They were exhibited in classrooms, at community theaters, and as part of professional training in mental health care education. As Kirsten Ostherr has argued, health films of all sorts (public health, individual health, and mental health) "were used everywhere, encompassing a wide range of topics concerned broadly with biopower, or the management of the self for the good of society."[5]

One such health film illustrates the genre's racial-pathologizing project. Funded by the US Department of Health, Education, and Welfare and produced for the National Institute of Mental Health by the Manhattan-based Ad Council, *A Day in the Death of Donny B.* was a fourteen-minute, one-reel film distributed to high schools with an accompanying teacher's guide for discussion. Figure 3.1 shows the film's title frame, in which a young Black man nods out from drugs in a doorframe on a city street, with cars and people passing him by.[6] Accompanied by the title's articulation of Donny B. as dying, this frame suggests congruencies among Black masculinity, the street, and death.

The film's narrative follows Donny, a young Black man, as he loiters on the streets of Harlem, nods out, hustles for money, tries (unsuccessfully) to steal, fends off dope sickness, then scores and shoots up in a ruined basement setting. These observational sequences of Donny are intercut with interviews where people talk about Donny or about addiction. Some of these people may be his friends; one woman says, "I know he's killing himself, and I have

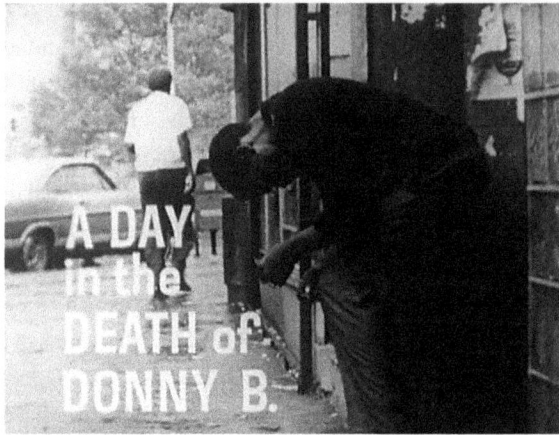

FIGURE 3.1. Title frame of *A Day in the Death of Donny B.* (1969).

a sneaking suspicion that he knows he's killing himself also." Others are state officials: A uniformed officer shows the prison cell where police lock up addicts; over shots of the city morgue, an off-screen voice presumed to be the city coroner discusses how the addict's life is one of social death. While some spoken words are diegetic, some of them accompany visuals of Donny, serving as commentary. Donny himself never speaks. A melancholy blues song plays for the film's fourteen minutes, with a repeating chorus, "Just another dirty ole day / in the death of Donny B."

The film employs cinéma vérité aesthetics; as Ostherr and others have noted, health and medical films made heavy use of aesthetics from avant-garde and experimental filmmaking, to the extent that some scholars, such as Lisa Cartwright, have asserted that medical films were imbricated with avant-garde modes of visuality.[7] In the case of *Donny B.*, I argue its cinéma vérité style served its public health promotional aims, granting it an aura of authenticity and "hipness" that would, in effect, "sell" it to those very audiences its narrative content pathologized.[8] Associated with "liveness" and "the real," cinéma verité aesthetics suggest that the short film is an addict's day in Harlem "captured in the making," not a fictional narrative scripted by the state. Its theme song grants it a hipness atypical to antidrug messaging, and it lacks the overarching narratorial voice (the [white male] "Voice of God") that often served the state documentary's authorizing function. Its aesthetics of the authentic, its hip bluesy theme, and its absence of a sonorous narrator code it as representing "voices of people," rather than of the state. In this, the film hides its state work of inculcating teenage viewers into proper (sober) citizenship.

Nevertheless, the film embodies sociological discourses that constructed the Black man as pathological, dangerous, and criminal; its formal silencing of Donny, who is literally without voice, representationally enacts sociological discourses in which "the Black man" was an object of study. Not insignificantly, the film codes Donny's failure to properly enact citizenship as queering him—a potential female romantic interest spurns him, and the pamphlet encouraged teachers to point out to students that men who used heroin lost their ability to sexually perform. This was typical of public health cinema more broadly, which connected proper citizenship to proper health practices to proper heterosexual relations, and it would reappear as well in *Hitch*.[9]

HITCH: MENTAL HEALTH FILMS DURING BLACK POWER

One motivation for producing *Hitch: Portrait of a Black Leader as a Young Man* was to promote the Northside Center for Child Development. Founded and directed by Black psychologists Kenneth and Mamie Clark, the center was located in Harlem. According to Markowitz and Rosner's detailed account of discussions among the center's administrators and staff, the center felt under pressure to respond to Black radicalism and its criticism of professional interventions.[10] Perhaps with these criticisms in mind, *Hitch*'s producer and director, Irving Jacoby, hired Black radical intellectual and artist Julian Mayfield to cowrite the script; letters between the two also indicate Jacoby attempted to hire crew from the local Black film production community. As discussed in chapter 1, Jacoby was an established mental hygiene filmmaker; he cofounded the Mental Health Film Board in 1949, which, in consultation with prominent midcentury psychologists and psychiatrists, produced more than fifty mental health films over the next twenty-five years. (It is likely that the Clarks contacted Jacoby through Viola Bernhard, who served on the Mental Health Film Board as well as the Northside Center's Board of Directors.) By hiring Mayfield and seeking out Black crew, Jacoby intended to craft a film whose production process, at least, honored Black radicalism and the local community.[11] Although the final cut of the film veered from Mayfield's early script versions, it contains a radical narrative remarkable for mental health filmmaking, including both explicit and implicit support of Black Power.[12] I will argue that its most radical impulses were, by its conclusion, muddled: The film's production was funded by a racial liberal philanthropic organization,

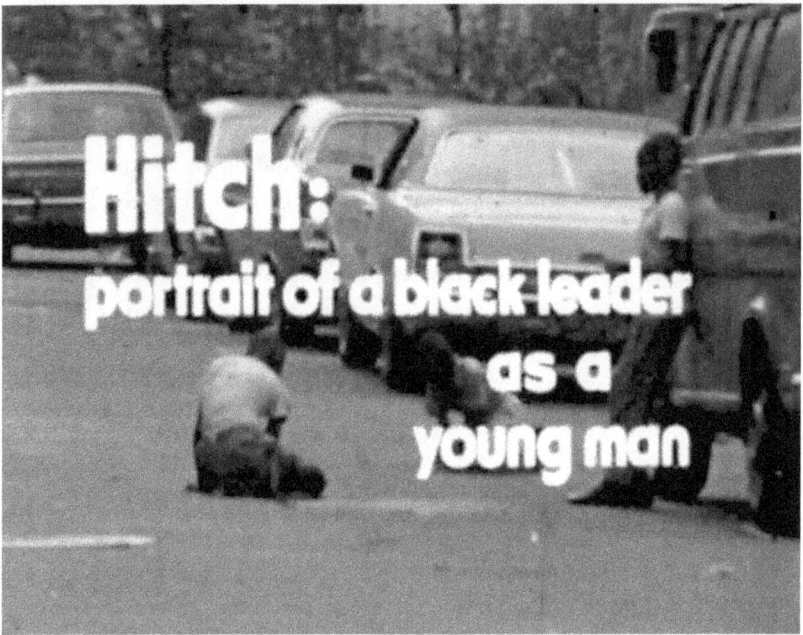

FIGURE 3.2. Title frame of *Hitch* (1971).

and the filmmaker would need more funding for additional distribution and exhibition, a constraint on just how radical it could be.

Sixteen-year-old Hitch, the film's protagonist, arrives in Harlem from South Carolina and soon makes two friends: Ricky, a streetwise sixteen-year-old who drops out of school, self-medicates with heroin, and goes to jail for six months; and Nevis, a bookish and unhappy girl. These three teenagers reside in the same tenement building with their different families: Hitch with his mother and grandmother, who await the imminent arrival of Hitch's father; Nevis with her mother and a father who ultimately leaves; and Ricky with his aunt and uncle, who sell bootleg alcohol and run numbers out of their apartment. With the rebellious Ricky as his guide to the city, Hitch tries out all it has to offer a young Black man, which it turns out, isn't much: He and Ricky hawk stolen LPs for a neighborhood black marketeer, who compensates them in marijuana; they find work at a midtown laundry, but the owner practices wage theft; and Hitch explores the possibilities for community transformation offered by the Black Panthers. Throughout the film, the three teenagers often return to discussing the lack of opportunities for children and young people, which is reflected in specific scenes and interlude shots depicting their impoverished school system and their lack of open green spaces to play. All three characters, particularly Nevis and Hitch, express a desire to find a way to help the community. Nevis, referred by school officials to the Northside Center for therapy, transforms, by the end of the film, into a happy young woman who organizes a tutoring program for the area's children. After Hitch's anger at racism manifests in a moment of violence, he transforms through the mentoring of his tenement's superintendent, Mr. Vance, and in the film's penultimate scene Hitch joins Nevis to lead a program that tutors children in Afrocentric history and culture, thus fulfilling the title's promise of a "Black leader." The final scene follows Hitch and Ricky as they walk through Harlem, Ricky having just been released from a sober six months in jail, and they talk hopefully about working to transform their community.

Produced at a time with an emerging cultural discourse that figured the "black male leader" through the supposed apposite dualism of Malcolm X as violent resistance and Martin Luther King Jr. as nonviolent resistance, the film is organized around answering the question implicit in its title (see figure 3.2, with the film's subtitle "Portrait of a Black Leader as a Young Man"): what kind of leader will Hitch become? Will an angry Hitch follow Ricky's path into a world of deviancy? Will he follow the Black Panthers' model of leadership? Or will he take a different route? A social realist bildungsroman, the film's narrative joins this question about leadership qualities to its naïve protagonist's exposure to the urban "ghetto." It drew as well on the era's teenage rebellion film, with one significant difference: It centered on a rebellious young Black man and on his psychological response to an absent Black father and matriarchal Black family structure.

Its first scenes set out the film's theme of absent Black fathers. As Mr. Vance shows the dilapidated apartment, where rodents can be seen running through cracks in the walls, to Hitch and his mother, he informs them that Hitch's father, whom they expected to meet there, has left for a job in Indiana. Fed up with his family, Hitch exits the apartment to the street, where Ricky blocks his path and confronts him. As other teenagers watch, Ricky verbally, then physically, roughs up Hitch. Hitch surprises him by wrestling him to the ground, which gains Ricky's respect and his acceptance by the other teenagers. Hauling a mattress up the staircase, Hitch meets Nevis, who asks why he's moved into "this dump"; when Hitch tells her his "daddy arranged it," Nevis says drily, "That figures." These opening scenes highlight a shared distrust of father figures, and they suggest Hitch fights in the street to express anger about his father's absence. Furthermore, Nevis's words imply that her father has disappointed her. Nevis's verbal skepticism of men, combined with her androgynous dress and hair, code her as queer. Queerness thus is linked to paternal failure.

When Hitch's father, Levi, eventually returns, he visits Vance in the tenement's basement. The two men catch up over drinks, and as Levi becomes visibly inebriated, he explains that since being laid off from his job he has worked as a trash collector. Embarrassed by his poverty and subsequent self-medicating, he hasn't been able to rejoin his family. "Well, hell, I was a good worker there. . . . Whatever I did, I did it hard. . . . But, hell, now I can't even work. . . . I'm good for nothing. Picking up junk is my speed, just about." As his face collapses in anguish, Hitch enters the basement, recognizes his father, and begs him to rejoin the family. Levi refuses, and the actor's face, tightly framed, reveals the depth of his distress and fatigue. The meeting precipitates a dark night of the soul for Hitch, who abjectly wanders the city's dark streets and, far from home, hails a cab, which bypasses him to stop for a white passenger. Furious, Hitch grabs the driver and beats him; on the verge of choking the man, Hitch runs off, ending back at Vance's, where Vance advises Hitch to find a way to channel his anger constructively.

In other words, the film mobilizes interconnected tropes of Black male pathology: the absent/failed (and deviant) father; the deviant young Black man whose deviancy arises from the father's absence. In particular, Hitch's assault on the driver reproduces cultural discourses, prevalent after the 1968 riots, of Black male violence. These tropes also parallel arguments made by Daniel Moynihan, in his influential Moynihan Report, that entrenched racial inequality derived from the so-called failure of the Black family structure to mirror that of white middle-class family structure.[13] The film also draws on what Moynihan identified as one site of Black familial pathology, the matriarchal family structure: Hitch's family unit comprises his mother and his grandmother, and Nevis's unit is herself and her mother.

In work about how the Moynihan Report and the public discussions it provoked encoded homosexuality as part of the report's infamous "tangle of pathology," Kevin Mumford argues that, although the report has since become identified as primarily critiquing matriarchal family structure, the report's actual more significant concern was the Black male as a deviant subject.[14] In the report, Moynihan describes the abjected Black man as "neurotic," "engaged in immature behavior," and "looking for instant gratification." Mumford convincingly argues that, read in its historical context, Moynihan's report coded this figure as queer. Taking Mumford's reading as a starting point, I will explore *Hitch*'s vexed deployment of tropes of pathology, which at once both attempted to de-pathologize these tropes at the same time that it reproduced "mental health" as linked to successful heternormativity.

The film explicitly narrates Hitch's reactions, Levi's situation, and Ricky's addiction as caused by their experiences of racism, capitalist labor and housing exploitation, and racist educational systems. In this, the film dilutes psychologizing and pathologizing discourses that either deployed or reproduced biological racist tropes. At the same time, Hitch's anger is framed as the failure of a proper Oedipal and white, middle-class family structure. In this sense, a psy-entific logic, and one that mirrors the Moynihan Report's general argument, orders the film's narrative. And, perhaps most importantly, Hitch and Ricky's relationship includes moments of possible homoeroticism, including when they peep through a window to watch a neighboring woman having sex and when they relax together on a rooftop getting high. The "tangle of pathology" seemingly surrounds and tempts Hitch.

Yet the film also includes alternatives to the white liberal interventions suggested by the report's focus on "fixing" the Black family. First, the film provides a substitute father figure in Vance. Second, the film represents the Black Panthers as an opportunity for young Black men to care for the community. Ricky and Hitch follow a group of children merrily running into a building, then observe them being cooked and fed breakfast by a Black Panther. Hitch says, "I thought they spent all their time shooting it out with the cops. What're they doing with kids?" Ricky responds, "That's part of their thing!" Hitch says he wants to think about joining them. As the audio track fills with the Panther leading the children in singing "Gimme that ole revolution!," the camera surveys an exterior wall filled with Black Power posters, zooming out to reveal it as the front of a Panther Party meeting space, from which Hitch exits—he has met with the Panthers to explore their work. This scene thus legitimates the Panthers as an organization delivering care to the community (rather than violently challenging the state) and, occurring early in the film, sets up the possibility that Hitch might become a Black leader in their style.

The film's concluding scenes show Hitch's evolution into a leader who provides care to children. After Hitch accepts Nevis's invitation to join her in her tutoring program for Harlem's children, both characters are shown reading to the children, leading them in martial arts and dance, and educating them about history—specifically, about Haiti and its self-governing, formerly enslaved people. The scene does not explicitly name what *kind* of school it is: Nevis calls it Time for Children, leaving its viewers to make extra-textual connections, if they have such knowledge, to recognize that its curriculum is not one Nevis and Hitch devised on their own but is modeled on the Black Panther Liberation Schools.[15] By leaving unnamed the Black radical nature of their curriculum, the film allows for different interpretations by different audiences. For some, it will be obvious that Hitch has integrated Panther teachings and is following in their path of leadership, becoming a Black radical leader. For others, Hitch and Nevis have become educators for their community, a less radical, more white liberal–friendly assumption of proper citizens engaged in the social reproduction of labor.

Here, the film evidences the tensions between the Black radicalism of the Panthers (and Julian Mayfield) and the racial liberalist stance of the film's financial backers. In 1967, Jacoby received an initial grant of $40,000 from the Grant Foundation, a philanthropic organization, and he needed an additional $80,000 to cover the film's entire budget. In late 1968, the Grant Foundation decided to provide the additional funding. In a letter to Jacoby, its director wrote, "The situation in Harlem and other ghetto communities is developing so quickly that time is a very important factor."[16] It is not entirely clear what the Grant Foundation assumed the film would do to address "the situation," but it is clear that a film promoting psy-services to urban youth appealed to the foundation as a means to address something—possibly the growing appeal, in 1968, of Black radicalism to young people. By the time of the film's initial exhibition in 1971, Jacoby promoted it with a press release that highlighted the racial liberal framing of art as a means to promote white people's sympathy: "There are six-million Black adolescents in America. To many Whites, this group is frightening and threatening. The film reveals Black adolescents as a source of strength and productivity."[17] The competing interpretations that its final scenes make available underscore that the film negotiated this conflicted terrain.

Even as the film was meant to promote the psychological services of the Northside Center, the center never appears; instead, Nevis discusses with Hitch her experiences with a white female therapist. When Hitch expresses skepticism about discussing one's feelings with a white lady, Nevis responds that while at first she felt similarly, she ultimately found the therapist trustworthy and felt better after their sessions. The film represents Nevis's psychological improvement through changes to her appearance: She starts wearing makeup, earrings, and more feminine clothing, and she plants a kiss on Hitch's cheek, sparking on his face an expression of romantic interest, after which Hitch joins Nevis in their heterosexual parental figuration as leaders of Time for Children. In other words, therapy heteronormalizes the previously queer-coded Black woman. Additionally, establishing Nevis and Hitch as heterosexual resolves the potential homoeroticism of Ricky and Hitch's relationship. In other words, because of therapy, Nevis ensures Hitch's entry into normative sexuality. We see here a very conventional psychiatric-inflected narrative about intervention into the queer pathological sexualities assumed in cultural discourses about the presumably pathological Black family and the nonnormative sexualities it presumably sparked. Therapeutic intervention reestablishes the heterosexual parenting unit.

SAM, SAM AND HARLEM:
DOCUMENTARY AESTHETICS FOR MUTUAL AID

With an understanding of how the normalizing logics of the psy-ences (both psychology and psychiatry) and their racial-liberal imperatives informed *Hitch*, we can turn now to the Black disability politics of *Sam, Sam and Harlem*. The visual metaphors embedded in terms often used to describe one cultural text's relation to another—"revisions" and "re-envisions"—are, in this instance, as material as they are figurative, because Sam Gaynor and Sam Walton literally watched the film crew shooting *Hitch*. Then, with their film, they revised its cinematic vision of Harlem. In a 1976 grant application for funding for their films, they implied this re-envisioning in an articulation of their cinematic philosophy: "[We Care films] often portray subjective conflict, a thematic core of expression of the community. There is no story or plot, in the conventional sense, rather a pictorial action piece with dramatic intensity and perception of the residents rather than [of] the film maker."[18] This philosophy of documentary—documentary as capturing "subjective conflict"—and its philosophy of community self-expression as multifarious subjectivities in conflict explicitly contests the implicit film philosophy of *Hitch*, where the filmmaker arrived on set with a preordained interpretation of the community hardened into the script, and where narrative logics worked to *resolve* conflict. I will argue that *Sam, Sam and Harlem* presented the community as self-determining, as engaged in its own expressions of conflict and methods of care that required neither resolution nor the state's intervention; rather than mobilizing formal logics of resolution or thematic instances of intervention, the film argues that expanding community-determined media productions is necessary for additional and continued expressions of conflict and mediation of methods of care. The film adds to our understanding of how Black activists used media to engage with Black disability activism and promote a widened Black public sphere.

Both Gaynor and Walton were community residents who volunteered, in the summer of 1968, to tutor children who visited the Clarks' Northside

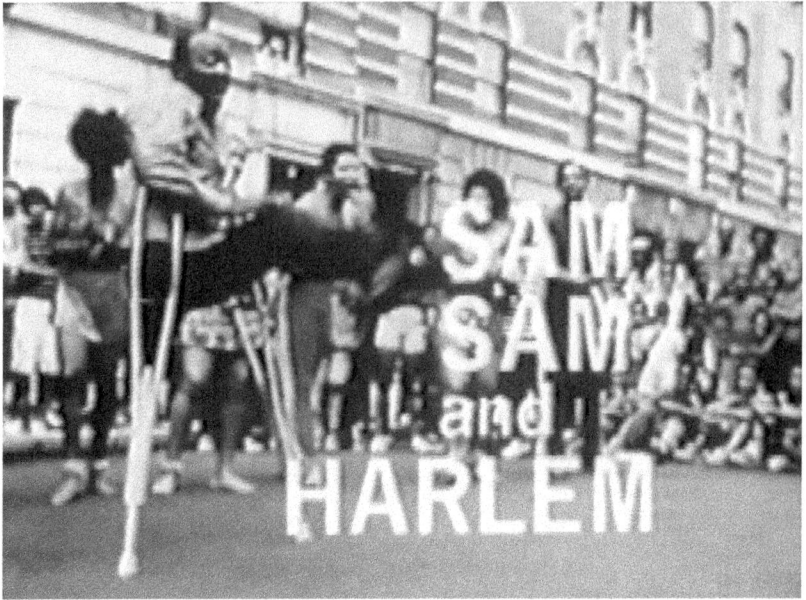

FIGURE 3.3. Title frame of *Sam, Sam and Harlem* (1974).

Center. Initially hesitant to engage nonprofessionals, ultimately the Clarks warmed to them and helped the young men, enlisting them for their tutoring services and vouching for them with funding agencies.[19] In 1971, Gaynor and Walton proposed developing a project for youth leadership in communications media and, from this, received, in 1973, limited technical support from the local ABC office as they wrote, directed, and produced the one-hour documentary about their activities as leaders of We Care.[20] It was broadcast in 1974 on the New York City ABC affiliate and shown to local Harlem audiences.

The film opens to a street fair, where young Black dancers, clothed in dance troupe uniforms, perform while drummers fill the air with rhythm. As a throng of onlookers cheers and sways, an older, one-legged man in everyday clothes enters the circle and, using his crutch for support, dances. In a freeze-frame, the film's title, *Sam, Sam and Harlem*, appears beside this dancing man (fig. 3.3). This title freeze-frame foregrounds that this is a signal theme of the film: community cultural expression on the streets.

Following this initial sequence, a male narrator talks about the topic often used by liberal reformers as evidence of "ghetto pathology"—violence in Harlem—in a rhetoric that de-sensationalizes it. Scenes of a funeral procession entering a church are accompanied by his words: "We had a shootout here last week, a black cop and two suspects dead." As a woman in the procession falls and another woman cries out "Momma, please stop crying," the camera cuts to four Black men, one looking at the camera, while the narrator says, "If you live in Harlem, you see a lot of that stuff." The heightened emotions of grief at a funeral are narrated with flat rhetoric, a rhetorical denudation of the affective import in public discourse about Black pathology typified in the trope of "Black-on-Black" violence. Credits appear identifying the narrator as Arthur French; his diction is colloquial, the rhythm of his words sparse, and the voice-over is distinct from the white diction typical of news documentaries of the time, embodied in voices such as Edward R. Murrow's.[21] The next scene follows two Black men through Harlem streets as they greet people and linger to look at street vendors' wares. As they wander, the narrator says that one can get an education on the streets of Harlem, "in drugs, crime, and some other things too," and that the film's two protagonists "dropped out of school when they were sixteen, and 125th Street was their college." The camera enters a bookstore, "the library for this college," and pans to the books displayed both on shelves on the sidewalk and in the store. The proprietor, Mr. Michaux, then explains that all the books in his store are about and by Black people, "save Webster's Dictionary." In this library, French narrates, Gaynor and Walton have read Black history, including Malcolm X, and it was after reading Malcolm X's printed words that they then went to his public appearances.[22]

With a voice-over that abjures the formal diction typical of broadcast news and public television documentaries as well as its theme of the street as place of education, the film grounds itself in a knowledge discourse distinct from that organizing mainstream representations of Black life, which relied on formal diction that evoked official social-scientific academic knowledge discourse that coded the ghetto as pathological. The vernacular, the quotidian, the street: These are generative of knowledge.

Multiple sequences establish Harlem streets as knowledge generating. From the bookstore as archive of knowledge and education, the film cuts to a sequence of public gathering spaces. This sequence begins first with a clip of Malcolm X, itself mediated (it appears to be a televised speech), who exhorts a Black audience to demand that the city fund Harlem schools. The film cuts to the streets of Harlem, where Black figures, each identified by caption, address crowds of people: Adam Clayton Powell Sr., surrounded by multiple microphones and reporters; Charles Kenyatta; Lucille Levy; and, finally, Pork Chop Davis. In cutting from Malcolm X's mediated event to these street scenes, the film emphasizes that a Black public sphere, electronically projected over either television in the case of Malcolm X or microphones and loudspeak-

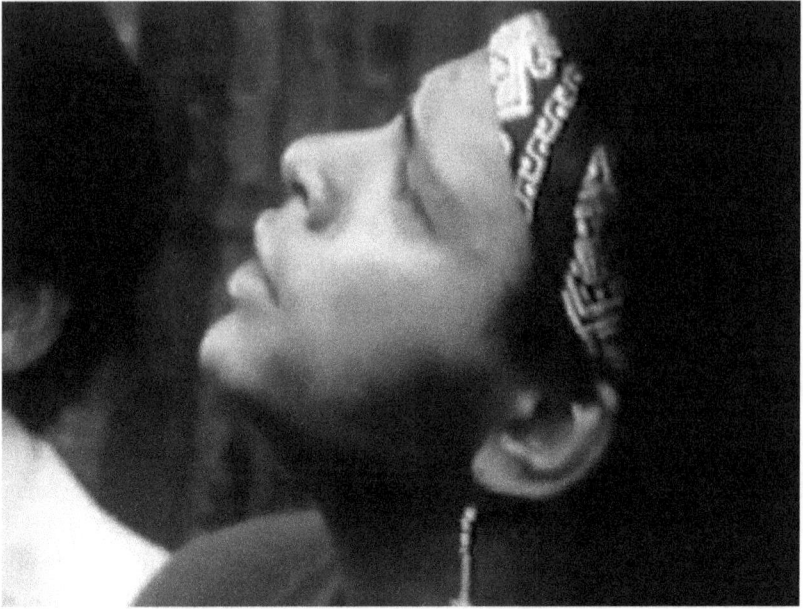

FIGURE 3.4. *Sam, Sam and Harlem* (1974).

ers in the case of Powell and others, exists *on the street*. Drawing from the documentary convention of identifying authorities through captions, the biographical captions included in these scenes establish these figures as Black authorities. Thus at the same time that this scene establishes Harlem residents and activists as authorities who circulate their own knowledge discourse, its form strips official discourse of its claims to truth reiterated in broadcast media.

Again shot on the street, scenes in which Gaynor and Walton speak with people experiencing addiction visually encapsulate an aesthetics of reciprocity.[23] Four Black men sitting on a stoop hail Gaynor and Walton. As the two groups of men begin speaking, the camera zooms in to a close-up on the seated speaker, who wears a bandana headband and a dangling earring (fig. 3.4). He speaks with a blunt, raw attitude, saying, "I hear you all got a little thang going on, doing a little help for somebody.... I'm out here man, I'm trying to get a little across, man, but I can't seem to get a play, man." The scene cuts to a midrange close-up of Gaynor and Walton crouched down on the sidewalk. Their eyes appear to be level to the man who is speaking, and they are listening intently to him (fig. 3.5).

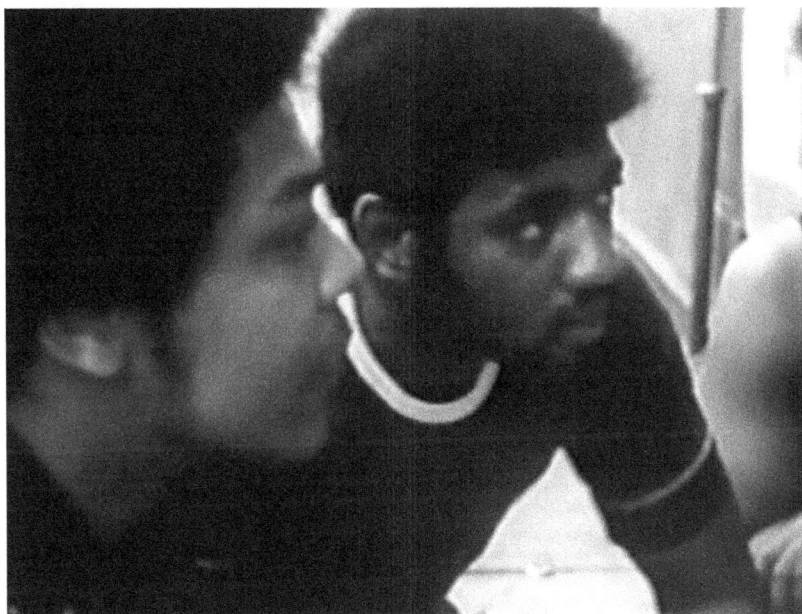

FIGURE 3.5. *Sam, Sam and Harlem* (1974).

All three men discuss the man's work history. He explains that he recently got out of jail and has been experiencing addiction for ten years. During this conversation, it is difficult to hear Gaynor and Walton; their voices are muted, the sound levels louder when the man experiencing addiction speaks.[24] This formal choice that diminishes Gaynor and Walton's words and amplifies those of the man experiencing addiction creates a reciprocity between the voice of the man and those who seek to care for him, and it resists the conventional formal devices in nontheatrical cinema that silence those with addiction in order to let the voices of the state speak about them—the formal silencing of the man experiencing addiction in *Donny B*. It contrasts with *Hitch* too, where Ricky and the addiction he experiences, while sympathetically depicted, is constructed within a narrative that encourages speculating about causes (Is it familial dysfunction? A poor educational system? A lack of opportunities?), rendering it a problem requiring psycho-sociological knowledge discourse. When the film cuts to a different location, Gaynor and Walton talk with a woman experiencing addiction who tells them that she keeps trying to enter a rehab program but is always told the program can't help her. The scene concludes with her words: "I mean, I need help!" The denial of desired care suggests she experiences medical racism and highlights state austerity policies toward Black communities.

In another scene, the two men counsel a woman standing in front of a parked car, cars passing by behind them. Their discussion centers on gathering information from the woman so that they can figure out how to direct her to work opportunities. This emphasis on care taking place on the street itself, realized in the continued mise-en-scène of the sidewalks and streets, foregrounds the community in the street as the site of locution, as producer of meaning. (This is not to say that there aren't scenes that take place in interior spaces—in fact, some do, but such scenes concern organizing efforts, which are different than the actualization of care shown in these other street scenes.) That meaning becomes legible once the media production is spatially embedded within the street itself. The film thus eschews the social scientific gaze of "the street" common in the 1940s photo-text style that Paula Massood notes dominated magazine representations of Harlem projects and that moved into cinema through the quasi-documentary *The Quiet One* (dir. Sidney Meyers; 1948), a gaze derived from the knowledge discourse of racial liberalist institutions and used for racial liberalist goals of engendering white people's understanding.[25] The film makes specific formal choices that divest "the street" of culturally hegemonic discourses; it stages itself—through its mise-en-scène, sound, and diction—as indexing Black knowledge. In doing so, its producers/subjects, Gaynor and Walton, articulated a documentary method that countered the genre's origins in ethnographic filmmaking, with its heritage of Othering its documentary subjects, as well as the genre of television documentaries about "problems of the urban ghetto" that championed social scientific discourses and liberalism, rendering "life on the streets" as a problem requiring liberal interventions.

In other words, in this film the streets produce and circulate Black education and knowledge, a circulation it tracks in its organization of scenes that move between exterior spaces and interior spaces and by describing communications media as the method by which such circulation can be accomplished. This is more than a flâneur style of filmmaking—the film is doing more than traveling and spectating: It intends its movement through the exteriors and interiors of Harlem to provide a route for the future media-makers the film aims to engender.[26] In a sidewalk scene, Gaynor and Walton talk to a single mother who needs help, the street serving as their office, and they discuss sending her to the Northside Center for counseling and work placement. Following this, an interior scene shows this young woman being introduced as a We Care summer worker to a switchboard operator; she sits and watches the operator explain how to work the switchboard. A side-angle close-up showcases her intensity, and when the switchboard operator's arm cuts through the frame to work the machinery, our attention is directed to the communications media on which the two people work. The care Gaynor and Walton provide on the street moves the woman from the street to learning how to operate communications media.

Subsequent scenes concern other We Care educational and tenant aid efforts, which culminate in scenes of community control of media. An audience of young Black people listens to social workers speak about how to enter the profession; this is followed by scenes showing a We Care office meeting, then We Care working for tenants by reporting to the city rat bites and helping tenants file documents with city bureaucracies. Then, the narrator states that, to improve the poor press coverage of Harlem, the Sams contacted United Press International, which furnished help; an interior scene shows a white journalist advising young Black people how to conduct interviews, and the next scene shows them, outside, using microphones to interview local residents. In other words, following scenes of young people being tutored in communications media (the switchboard), receiving educations in entering the caring professions, and We Care working to improve people's living conditions, the film climaxes with this scene of youths learning how to use mass communications to document their own community—practicing community control of representing Harlem.

The film then returns to a street, where children play hopscotch on the macadam, and Gaynor and Walton wander among them as they return, the narrator tells us, to their real education, "on the streets." This final scene shows people, including children, reading and circulating a newspaper with a headline about Harlem (presumably the one that We Care has produced). They encounter a sharply dressed man; the narrator says, "Sometimes, you just can't make your case." Gaynor and Walton ask the man if he would consider volunteering some time to help Harlem's children, and the man pushes one of the children out of his way as he struts off, saying, "I ain't got time for that.... I'm in a hurry." One of the Sams says, his tone dry and bemused, "I'll see you later, Frank." The children cheer as Frank speeds off in his Cadillac. While much about Frank—his mannerisms, his attitude; how the We Care group responds to him—suggests he might be schooled in the other kinds of education the film mentions (e.g., drugs), neither the narrator nor the Sams name him as a problem. Rather than drawing on sociological discourses that might label Frank an example or a symptom of urban pathology, the film conveys the community responding to him with irony and humor, and the suggestion that they will welcome Frank should he decide to join their work of mutual aid. Here we see a clear instance of Gaynor and Walton's documentary philosophy: "[We Care films] often portray subjective conflict, a thematic core of expression of the community." In other words, rather than elide this scene of Frank, a possible symbol of pathology, from the film, and rather than fit Frank into a narrative of deviancy, the film shows the varieties of conflict—multifarious subjectivities—happening on the street. In fact, that the film arrives at its conclusion with this scene, I would argue, highlights this conflict, which, as Gaynor and Walton state, is, to them, a "core of expression of the community." This is a theory of mutual kinship: not of subject and object, not of wielder of knowledge and object of knowledge, but rather of mutual subjective humans in kinship (and conflict) with each other.

The film ends with a scene that returns to the street festival that opened the film. The narrator says, "It's like Pork Chop Davis says: The black man has to get organized to help his own people; that's what We Care is all about!" As shown in figure 3.6, this time the one-legged Black man throws his crutch away, dancing on one leg as the people raucously cheer him on. Then, with another freeze-frame of his joyful figure, credits appear that thank the entire community for contributing to the making of the documentary.

In their history of the Northside Center, Markowitz and Rosner interpret this scene as a representational prosthesis, where the man no longer needs his "crutch" due to the power of We Care to "make able" the Black community.[27] This does seem one possible reading, especially when the scene is considered in relation to the narrator's words. Yet as Schalk argues, concepts from white disability studies, including narrative prosthesis, where race was not a constitutive underpinning of the conceptual framework, do not necessarily translate directly into racialized contexts.[28] In light of this, I want to consider other readings. The film concludes with the same street celebration that began the film. The conclusion has one significant difference from the opening scene: It is not followed by a cut to a funeral for a Black cop and two Black suspects. This return to the street celebration might thus be read as a reclamation of the streets for Black male joy, rather than showing the streets as places of mourning. It might also be read as a scene of an individual "overcoming" disability, or even as inspiration porn. We might also consider the ways in which the film at certain points centers Black men and Black manhood, and that this final visual scene, combined with a narration that centers Black men, might ges-

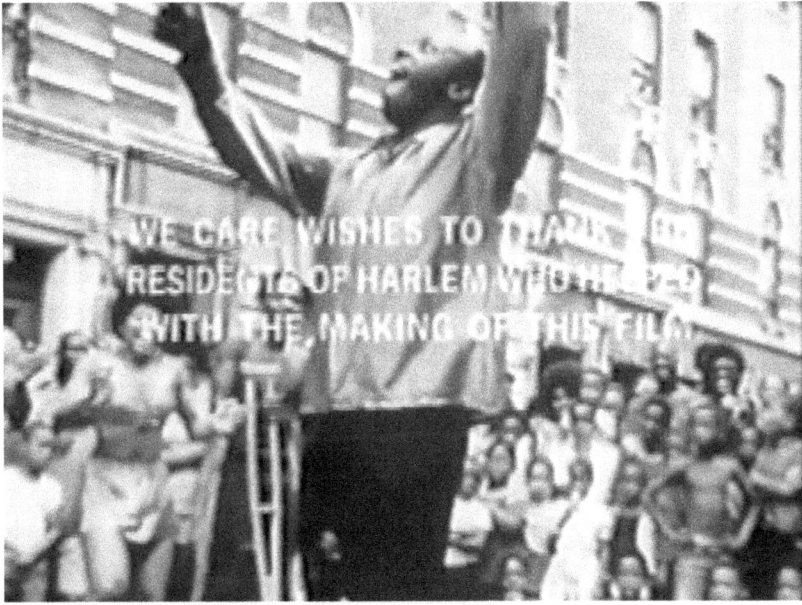

FIGURE 3.6. *Sam, Sam and Harlem* (1974).

ture toward what others have identified as weaknesses in social movements that failed to dismantle heteropatriarchy.[29] Yet if we consider that the man is surrounded by other dancers and musicians, perhaps we might read this as an invitation to think beyond conceptual categories of disability and ability, beyond mental health and mental illness. Perhaps the final dance remarks on artistic production itself as a form of mutual aid.

Conclusion

Gaynor and Walton's film should be contextualized within the broader media and technological landscape of 1973: the rise of a culture of information and informatics. With its multiple media and technologies, including the switchboard, the newspaper, and filmed interviews on the street, combined with its inclusion of We Care scenes documenting how the organization served as conduit between Harlem residents and city services, the documentary embeds communications media as integral to a Black-determined politics of information. That politics was exemplified in the newsletter, *City Scene*, that Gaynor and Walton produced and that expressly aimed to help Harlem residents with social services, health information, and understanding new city policies as they went into effect. In one grant application, Gaynor and Walton argued that *City Scene* would address the lack of a Black press that served Black residents, noting that a local Black paper was under heavy criticism for not serving its Black community. This was a form of information activism, of using print media to deliver vital information.

In *Crip Genealogies*, the coeditors note that the term "crip" is wielded in opposition to how "disability" has come to serve (racial liberal) bureaucracies and their resource-appointing and -diminishing functions.[30] It could be argued that, in acting as intermediaries between Black residents and city services—in some senses, in doing the work that the state would not do—Gaynor and Walton perhaps supported the state and its bureaucracies of racial liberalism. Yet reading their media production through the lens of Black disability studies refutes this. Theirs was a resistant practice. In their documentary, they resisted pathologizing tropes and aesthetics, including the rhetorical and aural expression of social scientific discourse typical of television documentaries about "the ghetto." They worked to construct a public sphere that could become self-sustaining in its mutual aid efforts, using whatever means available to acquire funding for a self-determined Black media and information ecosystem. They sought methods to make information available to all. Thus, I argue that we should consider the film they made Black disability media; we should also consider their entire project a form of crip-of-color information politics.

Jina Kim elaborates crip-of-color critique as mobilizing disability not as a noun but as a verb—drawing on Ruthie Gilmore's definition of racism, Kim defines this as "the state-sanctioned disablement of racialized and impoverished communities via resource deprivation."[31] At the time of *Sam, Sam and Harlem*'s production, the Urban Institute's Micro Analysis of Transfers to Households (MATH) microsimulation model was at the center of debates over welfare and food stamps in New York, making headlines as state agencies instituted "policy analysis" into their decisions.[32] By elucidating structures of interdependency and mutual aid arising to combat the state's practices of debilitation that targeted Harlem and its communities of color and by eschewing state-funded service provisions, Gaynor and Walton implicitly rejected the "sciences" involved in these decisions. Through a vernacular aesthetics that similarly countered the expert, social scientific–derived aesthetics of mental hygiene cinema, their re-envisioning of caring for people in distress through community-determined media was, in essence, a practice of mutual aid through cultural production.

Chapter 4 pursues in more detail how simulation, whether a datafied model or a mediated one, became a psy-entific technology of debilitation—and how feminist-of-color media production took up the threads of interlocking oppressions that the insurgent media discussed in this chapter might be said to have dropped. We move now from the streets, to the performative stage, and then to the kitchen table.

4

COUNTERING PSYCHIATRIC WAYS OF
SIMULATING/RACIALIZING PATIENTS

[In prison,] I had several sessions with a psychiatrist. His conclusion was that I hated my mother. How he arrived at this conclusion I'll never know, because he knew nothing about my mother; and when he'd asked me questions I would answer with absurd lies. What revolted me about him was that he heard me denouncing the whites, yet each time he interviewed me he deliberately guided the conversation back to my family life, to my childhood. That in itself was all right, but he deliberately blocked all my attempts to bring out the racial question, and he made it clear he was not interested in my attitude toward whites.—ELDRIDGE CLEAVER, *Soul on Ice*

As attendees of the 1969 American Group Psychotherapy Association conference watched, four influential New York psychiatrists, one after the other, conducted therapy with a working-class Black family composed of a grandmother, mother and father, and two children. When all four therapy sessions concluded, Dr. Clifford Sager brought the therapists back onstage, where they and the family members took questions from the audience. A few weeks later, each psychiatrist was informed that the Black family he had counseled was not a real family but instead made up of counselors from the

Partial Hospitalization Unit at Metropolitan Hospital, who had drawn from their interactions with working-class clients to perform as the family. The psychiatrists' reactions to this news and reflections about the event were taped. Transcripts of the event were published, alongside interviews with all participants, as a book, *Black Ghetto Family in Therapy: A Laboratory Experience*, by the countercultural publisher Grove Press in 1970. This chapter's epigraph, the Eldridge Cleaver quote, also served as the book's epigraph. The live event was videotaped, and in their introduction to the book, the event's organizers invited readers to request the videotape.

Thus far, that videotape remains lost, and so this chapter reads the event's archive through its print media. Even without access to that visual recording, I view the event as engaging a psychiatric way of screening, one that emerged during the Cold War era: simulating patients. Like other psychiatric ways of screening discussed in previous chapters, simulating patients performed two actions. First, it crafted as its object an imagined patient, often imagined as having excessive affective intensities or whose racial, class, or gender difference from the psychiatrist posed a threat. Second, it encoded those imagined differences into its operations, whether those were computational, videotaped, or live performances.

Like other psychiatric ways of screening, simulations responded to ongoing critiques of psychiatry as racist—in particular, critiques that psychiatry was failing to help working-class Black communities, but also, as in Cleaver's recounting, the inability of psychiatry to confront the politics of race, whether in the psychiatrist's office or in prisons. The simulation performed onstage at the conference—where Black professionals pretended to be a Black working-class family—was, for the event's organizers, ethically justified, because it protected the privacy of a real Black working-class family that participating in such an event would violate. However, the event's publication as a book by a countercultural press suggests a broader fascination with simulations of Blackness. Indeed, this was a common trope in the era's representational media. Journalist John Howard Griffin's *Black Like Me* (1961) and Grace Halsell's follow-up *Soul Sister* (1969), both bestsellers, recounted their white authors' experiences passing as black; Griffin's book also became a 1964 film. In 1967, William Styron's bestselling novel *The Confessions of Nat Turner*, in which the white author ventriloquized its black protagonist, provoked an edited collection of responses by Black writers, *William Styron's Nat Turner: Ten Black Writers Respond* (1968). Literary and cultural studies scholars have contextualized these performances of Blackness within histories of passing, where passing exposes the instability of naturalized categories of race.[1] In related work, Alicia Gaines argues that racial masquerade, where white people "wear" blackness for a day or more, exemplifies the racial liberal thematic of "cross-racial empathy and heroic whiteness."[2] While the performance of a Black working-class family at the 1969 conference did not involve racial masquerade, it nevertheless involved artifice: the simulation of the people of interest. Here, (white) psychiatry confronted its racist past and present through simulation.

Within psychiatric and psychotherapeutic research and training, simulations were positioned as creating a safe encounter with racial differences, ones that could both foster white psychiatrists' cross-racial empathy and confer cultural capital to psychiatry as finally, "heroically," overcoming its racist past. In the psychotherapeutic professions, this simulative logic cleaved to psychiatrists' energetic experiments with the emerging media of computers and portable video (already explored in chapter 1). In this chapter, I argue that media and technological innovations in medicine and psychiatry's simulated patients established a white, middle-class normate. Psychotherapists produced these innovations within the context of antipsychiatry discourses and the rise of alternative therapy, and, as I will show, they sometimes couched their innovations in response to these. But, as Elisabeth Lasch-Quinn argues, alternative therapy itself co-opted the moral energies of the Civil Rights Movement through a focus on individual, rather than social, political, and economic—that is, structural—transformation.[3] Through discussions of a documentary broadcast on PBS, William Greaves's *In the Company of Men* (1969), and *A Dream Is What You Wake Up From* (1978), a narrative film by Larry Bullard and Carolyn Johnson, members of the radical filmmaking collective Third World Newsreel, I demonstrate that Black cultural production wrestled with this co-optation. In their creative works, Black media-makers pushed against psychotherapeutic uses of simulation, critiquing them as a technology of racializing pathologization. Although Greaves's film took up simulative practices for the liberal project of soothing strained racial and class relations, it revealed white men's emotional capacities to be more pathological than those of Black men, and thus as de-pathologized Black men by showcasing their flexibility with the "emotional loosening up" that was coming to the cultural fore. Bullard and Johnson more directly deconstructed simulation in psychotherapeutic practices as a means of reproducing class differences and gendered oppression. In other words, Black media-makers critiqued the psy professions' naive use of simulation, illuminating it to be a tool that naturalized class, race, and gender oppression.

Cultures of Simulation: A Short History

Psychotherapeutic simulation drew from a broader Cold War culture of simulation. Technological simulation arose out of Norbert Wiener's work promoting the cybernetics paradigm and the US air defense's SAGE (Semi-Automated Ground Environment, spearheaded by the think tank RAND Corporation). As Paul Edwards has shown, SAGE created the close to one thousand technical experts who would become preeminent figures in the programming field, having learned, among other skills, SAGE's simulation techniques meant to prepare for a thermonuclear battle between superpowers.[4] Simulations quickly bled from the military-industrial complex into the management industries and academic disciplines. By 1969, economics, the biological sciences, management, the social sciences, education, political campaigning, and psychology accepted simulation as research methodology and for applied contexts.[5] A 1972 volume on simulations defended them as methods for theory-building, experimenting, and teaching.[6]

A nonexhaustive list of simulations for race-related topics illuminates the basic drive to govern racialization through simulation. Social scientists developed a computer simulation that used economic variables from 1960s census records to predict factors that might lead to racial equality by 1990.[7] In another project, sociologists used computer simulations of racial discrimination in racially segregated housing.[8] In college and K–12 classrooms, sociologists used a game, GHETTO, to teach "non-ghetto" residents about "ghetto" residents, exemplifying how simulations took up the liberal cause of stimulating cross-racial empathy.[9] But these simulations that bled from the military to urban imaginaries were not mere abstract exercises in pedagogy or theory-building. As Jennifer Light documents, in Pittsburgh, city planners applied to their projects of urban renewal the outcomes of their computer simulations.[10] Alice O'Connor argues that, beginning in the late 1960s and stretching beyond the Reagan administration, microsimulation became standard practice in the think tank–sponsored research-and-policy nexus, with immediate effects on policymaking, in particular how resources would be apportioned to impoverished communities.[11] Simulations, then, were racializing projects.

In the psychotherapeutic domains, three types of simulations dominated this decade: psychodrama; videotaping of simulated patients; and computerized simulations of patients. Psychodrama was invented by Jacob L. Moreno (also discussed in this book's introduction). An advocate of improvisational theater as active and a critic of the psychoanalytic couch as passive, Moreno envisioned psychodrama, which placed bodies and minds in a highly structured event, as a "science of action."[12] In psychodrama, participants were assigned roles to play. In some cases the participant enacted the character of the person they were role-playing with; in other cases they pretended to be a person causing them psychological troubles (e.g., a mother). In other words, this "science of action" was also a simulation.

Moreno used psychodrama at Sing Sing Prison, the Hudson Reformatory, and his own Hudson Valley institution founded in 1936, and it quickly spread after World War II as a method for veterans. Saint Elizabeths in Washington, DC, built a dedicated stage for psychodramas.[13] Another Moreno invention, sociodrama, was psychodrama's group relations version, intended to address "negative relations" within society. After World War II, the state employed sociodrama to defuse tense racial relations.[14] By the 1960s, Moreno's psychodrama and sociodrama merged with the cultural zeitgeist of encounter-group therapy and other human potential movement precursors. Organizations trained psychodrama facilitators who could lead sessions for corporate executives.[15] (We shall see this background take form in Greaves's *In the Company of Men*.)

As psychodrama filtered into countercultural and mainstream practices, videotape entered the area of psychotherapeutic simulation.[16] By the 1960s researchers considered videotaped simulated patients an adequate way to avoid the ethical quandaries of allowing trainee counselors to interact with real patients. As one of them put it, videotaping a simulated therapy client enabled "maximum control of the counseling student-client interaction for desired objectives [that will prevent] harmful effects to the client."[17] The collision of videotape with simulation in psychotherapeutic domains hit a high point in the early 1970s: Clinical psychology professors had students simulate patients and staff of a mental institution and videotaped it for research purposes, and supervisors at Elgin State Hospital used a three-day weekend to run a mock mental ward where staff "played" being patients, again videotaping the entire event for future review.[18] (The most famous exercise in simulating psychiatric patients, the Rosenhan Experiment, reversed these two examples by introducing simulated schizophrenics into real mental hospitals.)

At the RAND Corporation, researchers sought to computerize the psychiatric training process. Richard Bellman, who worked at Los Alamos before joining RAND, developed a computerized initial psychiatric interview meant to augment psychiatric training.[19] Explicit about his model's roots in the military-industrial complex, Bellman wrote that "situations of complexity and uncertainty comparable to those encountered in a psychiatric interview are fairly common in the business and military spheres, and here the technique of mathematical simulation has spurred much insight."[20] For Bellman, the therapeutic session contained an "information pattern," upon which "decisions are made," which produce "events" that then influence "the information pattern," and thus there is "a 'feedback' process."[21] In other words, Bellman aimed to apply the command-and-control logic of cybernetics and the US military to the affective domain of the psychiatric interview. His work at RAND, where employees programmed military simulations, was perhaps what inspired his almost-psychopathic choice of name for his computerized therapist—Dr. Strangelove. (This name was elided in the 1969 peer-reviewed publication of this research in *Computers in Behavioral Science*, which renamed therapist Dr. Strangelove simply "the therapist."[22])

In his attempt to make mathematical the interpersonal, unruly, and affectively laden interactions of a therapist and client, Bellman helped to embody the cybernetic communications logic of this era, where information "lost its body" and social relations were made modular within the logic of code.[23] Additionally, Bellman's project builds on the postwar intensification of earlier decades' moves to standardize medical training. In the case of programmers who developed patient computer programs, their work inevitably included a justification that computation would become a necessary skillset within academic medicine. These moves, as Moya Bailey and others have argued, accompanied widespread social and demographic shifts within medicine. They deployed standardization in order to assert white medical authority and construct the standard doctor as a white man with elite educational training.[24]

Other simulated psychotherapeutic patient programs constructed their client as a normate white man. In 1973, Thomas Hummel developed CLIENT 1, a simulated patient computer program for use in counselor training. CLIENT 1 was a thirty-year-old man "who is reasonably verbal and motivated and who is not overly resistant to describing his concerns to a counselor who[m] he can trust" and is conversant on the topics of work, family, and relationships with others.[25] Unremarked by the authors is the simulated patient's heterosexuality: The central conflict of one "conversation" in the included programmed responses concerns his aroused feelings when he encounters a female secretary. When Hummel published an expanded version of this report in a 1984 special issue of a counselor training journal about computers as counseling and training tools, the example client remained the same: a thirty-year-old, racially unmarked, and therefore white, heterosexual man.[26]

The research on videotaped and computerized patients of this period fails to identify simulated patients' race unless they are specifically Black, highlighting that the presumed normate for simulated patienthood was a white patient. Conversely, when racialized Blackness was identified, it signaled that the presumed normate for the psychotherapeutic professional was white, or someone who could conform their affects to the registers expected by psychotherapeutic training protocols and thus the psychotherapeutic habitus. In other words, Blackness was constituted as a vexing problem of affect, both of the patient who was too affective and for the trainee who must learn to comport themselves through racialized codes of professional affective behavior.

In her work, Kelly Underman argues that the standardized (and simulated) patient is a technology of affect. This technology trains students into their professional habitus and its affective demeanor. Because the standardized patient program is also a mode of assessment (the standardized patient has a checklist to evaluate the trainee), the technology transforms affect into scientific values of objectivity and measurement.[27] The technologies I discuss here lacked a version of the "checklist," although by the 1970s simulated therapeutic encounters started to incorporate feedback from actors. The technologies did, however, clearly seek to govern professional affect. For example, the author of "Training Counselors Through Simulated Racial Encounters" hypothesized that videotaped vignettes of "Black people in the ghetto" would be more efficient at addressing counselors' learned racism than sensitivity training would be. He wrote, because "Black pride and solidarity have 'set' Black clients to overreact and/or be on guard with white counselors," with vignettes, counselors could practice responding without "personalizing the experience" and could do so in a setting with "no possibility of harming clients."[28] For these vignettes, the author hired young Black people of unspecified gender to simulate clients. The actors were filmed delivering a monologue in which they expressed negative emotions; these were then watched by trainees, who were instructed to identify the simulated clients' affects. Trainees would then discuss with their advisor their own emotional reactions. In this setting, Blackness is constructed as intransigent, a problem, and counseling a young Black person is marked out as a "racial encounter." This "vexing" client produces dangerous affective responses in the trainee, whose affective responses must be disciplined into a proper affective comportment. A taped and simulated patient becomes a screen that reinforces boundaries between the therapist and the client, that allows the therapeutic, through its encounter with the unreal, to assert its professional authority to address a perceived real. What we see coalescing in this 1960s and 1970s psy-media-technological research on simulated patients is a template for the "normate" of simulated psychiatric patienthood. That normate was white.

Much of the published work of this period evidences an anxiety over the similarities among simulation, psychodrama, and deceptiveness or artificiality. This anxiety is evident among those working with technological simulations, for example, Kenneth Colby, who in his 1964 article "Experimental Treatment of Neurotic Computer Programs" wrote, "As a technical term, the word 'simulation' is perhaps an unhappy choice since it is easily confused with everyday language usage, connoting the negatively evaluating synonyms of feigning or sham pretending."[29] This anxiety also clearly bothered psychotherapists; in his 1966 guide *Role Playing in Psychotherapy*, Raymond Corsini included this prefatory "Note on Terminology": "The term roleplaying has four connotations: 1. theatrical, wherein players . . . simulate . . . for the purpose of entertainment; 2. sociological, or patterns of behavior as dictated by social norms; 3. dissimulative, or deceptive behavior . . . ; and 4. educational, whereby people act out imaginary situations for purposes directed to self-understanding. . . . When used in psychotherapy, roleplaying falls in the last category."[30] In an era of heightened paranoia, McCarthyite redbaiting, Senate investigations into the Minnesota Multiphasic Personality Inventory, and, of course, patients like Eldridge Cleaver who deceived their prison psychiatrists, it is perhaps not surprising that professionals advocating for simulation and role-playing took pains to distance their practices from deceptive behavior. Perhaps the deception that was inherent to psychiatry—its fundamental ignorance of what constitutes "mental illness"—required such painstaking throat-clearing.

Building on Foucault's concept of "biopower," Jackie Orr offers "PSYCHO-power" as naming the "technologies of power and technologies of knowledge developed . . . to regulate the psychological life, health, and disorders of individuals and entire populations."[31] While other theorists that Orr draws on, for example, Nikolas Rose, offer related models, Orr's neologism—where this form of biopower is PSYCHOtic—better indicates that these related techniques, which run from Bellman's computerized training to the videotaped simulation of "racial encounters," of abstraction, standardization, simulation, and objectivity are enraptured with, engulfed in, the psychoses they simulate. The techniques provoke the very conditions that they claim are simply under study. As Orr puts it, "Playing seriously with the logistics and illogics of perception, PSYCHOpower may operate not only in the field of rationalizing techniques but in the form of magical appearances or the persuasive trick."[32] We turn now to one such trick.

Simulative Logics, Race, and the "Laboratory Experience"

Black Ghetto Family in Therapy: A Laboratory Experience documented an event in which four psychiatrists, before an audience of approximately two hundred and fifty people, counseled a simulated Black family.[33] Published in 1970, two years after the 1968 staging of the event, its distribution in book form suggests its authors thought it might reverberate beyond its original audience of therapists, serving as an exculpatory document for a profession embattled by criticisms wielded by the Black Panthers (as well as by Black psychiatrists) that psychiatry was profoundly racist. Indeed, the book's opening epigraph, a passage critical of psychiatry taken from *Soul on Ice* by Black Panther Eldridge Cleaver, suggests exculpation as the book's broadest goal. Locally, the book sought to reveal the profound difficulties that arose in psychiatric approaches to working-class Black families, because, as its coauthors explain in the book's opening, the "bold new approach" called for by John F. Kennedy and instantiated in the community mental health center movement was failing its charge of helping those in impoverished neighborhoods. By its concluding section, its authors used the event as evidence that white therapists must examine themselves and their responses to Black clients as "subjective responses . . . based on racist concepts," that white therapists must come to "a deeper knowledge" of the black family "through the crucible of friendship," and that the profession must include greater numbers of Black psychiatrists.[34] Its conclusion thus combined both a racial liberalist stance—the Black radical critique of psychiatry was captured by a reformist racial liberal stance that white psychiatrists must flush out their racist biases—and an integrationist stance focused on inclusive hiring. As Dennis Doyle has argued, this racial liberal stance by New York psychiatrists was, by 1970, common.[35] Meanwhile, its authors also emphasized that social conditions, not psychological issues, might be the real source of problems for Black impoverished families.

In other words, the conclusions its authors drew did not substantially diverge from other racial liberal recommendations circulating at the time about addressing racist psychiatry, and they also incorporated social psychiatry models that de-pathologized Blackness. Where the book did stand out among its intellectual brethren was in its provocative staging of simulated Black patients while the psychiatrists were kept in the dark about the simulation—at least, most of them, as I discuss. For the reader of the text (and perhaps for the attendees at the conference), this becomes the narrative "hook," the mystery that propels the reader forward—will any of the psychiatrists realize they are counseling actors? What kind of dramatic climax might that provoke? In his brief introductory remarks to the audience, Dr. Sager, described in the book as the "laboratory chairman," explains that the family is a simulated one, without further details. In the book, these remarks are preceded by a longer prefatory note that explains why and how the event happened, identifies the four psychiatrists' ethnicity (one Jewish, one Black, two white), and explains that the four actors of the family were social workers at the Partial Hospitalization Program and the Family Treatment Program at Metropolitan Hospital. It also informs readers that one of the psychiatrists already knew these social workers, but it does not identify which one.

With the preface having tuned the reader in to this narrative mystery, the question of truth versus simulation hovers throughout the text. The session transcripts are meant to render an objective textual translation of the event; they even contain parenthetical interjections ("*Laughter*"; "*angrily*") that, the authors tell us, the transcriptionist included from viewing the videotape. This assertion of objective fidelity to truth within the medium of print was, I think, meant to mirror the so-called objective fidelity to truth that the videotape recording would have produced. In this era, videotape was becoming part of scientific mechanisms for the production of evidence, and clearly the book's coauthors sought to reproduce within the affordances of textual publication that evidentiary-ness. Other small details seek as well to polish the book with psy-ence's sheen; for example, in their acknowledgments the authors identify the National Institute of Mental Health grant that funded the event.

At the same time, an apparatus of simulation—rhetorical, formal, and thematic—punctures this truth discourse at every turn. The book's opening quotation from *Soul on Ice*, which sets out the Black radical critique of psychiatry, is itself a description of simulation. Cleaver describes his prison sessions with a psychiatrist, "[whose] conclusion was that I hated my mother. How he arrived at this conclusion I'll never know, because he knew nothing about my mother; and *when he'd asked me questions I would answer with absurd lies. . . .* What revolted me about him," Cleaver writes, "was that he heard me denouncing the whites, yet each time he interviewed me he deliberately guided the conversation back to my family life, to my childhood. That in itself was all right, but he deliberately blocked all my attempts to bring out the racial question, and he made it clear he was not interested in my attitude toward whites" (emphasis added).[36] Thus, embedded in this critique of psychiatry's willing indifference to racism sits Cleaver's testimony that his psychiatric sessions unfolded around his own simulation of patienthood, a Black man agentially dissimulating in order to play the psychiatrist for a fool and escape psy power. Another framing device references simulation: The authors end their preface with a quote from Shakespeare's *Hamlet*: "The play's the thing / wherein I'll catch the conscience of the King." This reference to what is arguably the West's Ur-text, one also significant in Sigmund Freud's corpus, and that mobilizes a core psychoanalytic concept of guilt, underlines the dramatic, simulative, and psychoanalyzable qualities of what is to come. Formally, the book echoes stage plays: In addition to the stage play–style expressive descriptions (such as *"Laughter"* and *"deep sigh"*), at the beginning appears a list of the "family members" and a diagram of where people sat on the stage, reminiscent of stage-play instructions for directors. The *Hamlet* quotation's reference to conscience and guilt signals, or provokes, a psychoanalytic reading of the "play" as a method of exposing "the King's"—read: psychiatry's—crimes (of racism).

With this dramaturgical framing of the text, and knowing that one of the four psychiatrists (but which one?) was in on the trick, a reader approaches the session transcripts primed to receive moments of simulation and dissimulation, moments of *exposure of the simulative logics*. Whatever transpires during a session, the reader's attention returns to the trick itself. Sager notes, in the prologue, that details of each psychiatrist's ethnicity are salient for understanding the sessions—that two are white, one is Jewish, and one is African American. That salience manifests in the session led by Thomas Brayboy, the Black psychiatrist.[37] Within minutes of meeting, the daughter says, "[Dr. Brayboy] is a member. He knows," to which Brayboy responds, "I even know how to play the dozens."[38] This winking moment of a shared cultural idiom appears to put the family members at ease; they seem to open up more with Brayboy than with the previous psychiatrists. It is not until a later part of the book, in sections that transcribe post-event interviews with the four psychiatrists, that the true significance of "playing the dozens" reveals itself. In Brayboy's interview, he states that he recognized the people acting the roles of the family members: they were staff at a clinic where he often worked. In other words, when Brayboy entered the stage and the audience presumed the shared connection between the Black psychiatrist and the simulated working-class Black family concerned their shared Blackness, Brayboy himself not only recognized the truth of the situation but communicated to the actors that they were all "playing the dozens," engaging in a verbal signifying game among themselves.

While the book's preface, post-event interviews, and concluding section engage in the gravitas of academic discourse and its attempts at fidelity to the truth imply a scientific perspective, the entire endeavor seems completely far out. Readers will find their eyebrow muscles tested. Pushing boundaries, being "far out," I argue, was intentional: Its authors sought to align it with the counterculture and with the flourishing alternative therapeutic movement. The book's subtitle, *A Laboratory Experience*, is the first indication that the book pushes boundaries. Its description as a "laboratory" echoes Moreno's emphasis on psycho- and sociodrama as "science in action," but as a laboratory *experience*, the subtitle quite clearly evoked a broader countercultural discourse of "experience." The Jimi Hendrix Experience had infamously asked, via their 1967 album, *Are You Experienced?*, and in *The Politics of Experience* (1967), R. D. Laing, iconic figure of the counterculture, had defined madness as a kind of wisdom and, rhetorically, joined "experience" to his own antipsychiatric practices and thought. Naming *Black Ghetto Family* an *experience* gave it a countercultural aura that suggested it belonged to a "loosened-up" psychiatry, to use the term sociologist Sam Binkley views as a governing logic of this time.[39]

In formally mirroring a dramatic script, the book also alluded to Moreno's psychodrama. By the late 1960s, psychodrama, and its cousin, the encounter group, had become cemented in popular culture as countercultural, and, indeed, Sager sometimes refers to the simulators as "role-playing," which both underlines the countercultural orientation of the event and supports my claim that role-playing and simulation bled into each other. The book's publisher, Grove Press, specialized in modernist and avant-garde theater and literature, having published, by that time, the works of Samuel Beckett and Harold Pinter, and it had been sued on obscenity charges for publishing D. H. Lawrence's *Lady Chatterley's Lover*. Framed by an intertextual referentiality typical of modernist literature, the book calls to an audience primed to interpret it as a literary artifact—the very kind of literature in which its countercultural publisher specialized. Grove also published popular psychology texts (Eric Berne's 1964 bestseller, *Games People Play: The Psychology of Human Relationships*) as well as the English translation of Frantz Fanon's *Black Skin, White Masks* in 1967. In sum, Grove Press's market already covered psychiatry, social issues, and the literary—an educated readership that aligned itself with, whether or not they participated in, countercultural formations.

At the same time, the "experience" was also an addition into dominant paradigms of psy practice, namely the burgeoning arena of family therapy. Nathan Ackerman, an influential figure in that field, was part of the event. His participation situates the videotaping of the event within the longer psy-research practice of making interpersonal relations observable, even measurable, through the presumed "truth" of them that videotape and its playback features enabled. As Deborah Weinstein has so thoroughly documented, in the Cold War rise of family therapy, which transformed the individual-oriented mode of psychoanalysis into the group-oriented mode of family therapy, the issue of observability loomed large.[40] No longer was the therapeutic process a matter of dreams, the unconscious, or unresolved emotional tensions. Instead, researchers, influenced by systems theory, sought to change dynamics of relating among members of a family, who were thought to constitute a system. At the same time, researchers needed to build knowledge about the family system itself. Weinstein argues, "Researchers had to identify what they considered the significant facets of family life and how such things were knowable; in other words, the objects of their studies and their observational methods for gaining knowledge about those objects had a multifaceted and intertwined relationship, even if not explicitly articulated."[41] For Ackerman, these observational methods were best pursued, he argued, using "sound tape, closed-circuit TV, and motion picture" in family therapy.[42] Ackerman and other researchers in family therapy during these decades filmed, videotaped, and used one-way mirrors as technologies by which family systems could be recorded and observed, their truths unveiled. The influential Ackerman Institute for the Family, still active today in New York, housed and still houses multiple films of families in therapy, continuing its investment in technologies of recording and exhibition as methods for knowledge production and pedagogical training.

Yet observational recording practices of family therapy did not often—if ever—center Black families. Again, family therapy, like other therapeutic methods, was defined through a psy normate of whiteness—and how else could it have been, given "the family" was always already constituted as the white middle class, and Black families always already designated an impossibility within both the (Western) grammar of psychoanalysis, psychiatry, and sociology and the American grammar of Blackness as nonhuman? Thus the real provocation offered through this laboratory experience was that it placed "the Black family," that lodestar figure in cultural and professional discourses of American pathology, at center stage. In producing observable video of the simulated Black family undergoing therapy, its authors drew on the general psychiatric disciplinary enthusiasm for videotaping simulated patients. That I have not been able to recover this video from the archives of this era suggests, perhaps, that another generation identified it as a gimmick easily read as buttressing the critique of psychiatry as racist.

Simulative Logics, Race, and Broadcast TV:
In the Company of Men

As the "laboratory experience" took place at a Manhattan Hilton hotel, Black filmmaker and television producer William Greaves used Moreno's sociodrama method in a documentary sponsored by *Newsweek* magazine and broadcast on PBS. *In the Company of Men* (1968) showed white automobile-manufacturing plant foremen and unemployed Black autoworkers engaged in the simulative practice of role-playing for the purposes, as the narrator stated it, of sensitivity training—fostering in the managers an understanding of how workers experienced how the foremen treated them, with the goal of improving employer-employee relations to help the workers, now part of the "hardcore unemployed," rejoin the workforce. That PBS would broadcast this updated version of an earlier decade's deployment of sociodrama to defuse tense race and class relations exemplifies the broad cultural interest in modalities of simulation, psychotherapeutic practices, and media. Reading it in relation to *Black Ghetto Family*'s role-playing illuminates the cultural and psy-professional reach of simulative practices for matters of social import, especially those that elite discourse crafted as problems, in this case the Black working class. As the documentary bounces between supporting racialized class relations through its therapeutic mode and exposing the burden of and creativity emanating from Black men's double consciousness, it illuminates how, in the hands of a Black producer, mediations of simulative practices contained countertherapeutic opportunities unforeseen by psychiatry.

In a 1970 *New York Times* article, Greaves made the case for what he called "encounter television" as a means to address the "disease" of racism.

> By putting members of each [racialized] group before a set of television cameras, and geographically removing them from each other, we introduce a safety factor. Under these "sanitized" conditions, it would be possible for such groups to go after each other hammer and tongs, no holds barred! They can call each other all kinds of dirty names without the danger of actually doing physical violence to each other. The theatrical, not to mention the mental health dividends that would accrue from such encounters on television would be incalculable.... Obviously, there are those who would use the opportunity for strictly propaganda purposes, but the logic and the techniques of psychodramatic encounter are such that these purposes would be quickly eroded and what would be left would be men and women communicating.

Here Greaves evinced a conventional belief that a public sphere allowed citizens to engage in communicative acts that could restore civic relations. In the next paragraphs, Greaves echoed Herbert Marcuse's psychoanalytic understanding of the oppressions of the United States.

America is caught in the grip of myriad neurotic and psychotic trends. Call these trends racism, sexism, chauvinism, militarism, sadism, what you will. The fact remains that it is virtually impossible to develop the necessary number of psychiatrists, psychologists, analysts, therapists, and the like to cope with America's emotionally disturbed population. The concept of television group encounter, patterned after the inter-personal encounters which take place at such organizations as the Moreno Institute... offer a stop gap mechanism to arrest the deteriorating social diseases which are presently eating away at American society. Using the techniques of 20th century communications, we are now in a position to put the rednecks of Alabama in a direct encounter with the Black militants of Harlem, either on public or closed-circuit television. This is but one way to help America achieve mental health.... Of course, the big question is, can this kind of programming surface from the present flood of video trivia, or will it have to wait upon the courage of some forward thinking programmer in 1994?[43]

A full instance of Greaves's "encounter television"—its description so evocative of the internet—would not materialize until 1988, when Greaves himself produced such a documentary, *The Deep North*.[44]

The *New York Times* article was published six months after *In the Company of Men* was broadcast; perhaps the six film festival awards the documentary won influenced Greaves's desire to articulate, in the US newspaper of record, that such staged encounters could benefit society.[45] But I am not as sure as Greaves seems to be in this article that his encounter documentary, by putting "both sides" into direct, albeit mediated, contact, achieves "mental health," by which he seems to mean an alleviation of racial struggle through parity, a both-sides-ism. In his illuminating article on Greaves's two sociodramas (*In the Company of Men* and *The Deep North*), filmmaker J. J. Murphy convincingly argues that a therapeutic imperative drove Greaves's sociodramas.[46] And so, reading against the grain of both Murphy and Greaves himself, I will argue that *In the Company of Men* achieves something Greaves either didn't or couldn't articulate: Within the counterculture-inspired rise of emotional expressivity as valuable and core to therapeutic endeavors, his documentary exposed white middle-class men as inflexible, and in doing so it deconstructed some of the underlying assumptions on which psychiatry's edifice of racialized pathologies was built.

The film was financed by *Newsweek* with the cooperation of General Motors Corporation and International Telephone and Telegraph, as well as three organizations: the Opportunities Industrialization Center, the Moreno Institute of Psychodrama, and the Jackson Cultural Institute. Set in a seminar room filled with desks, the film brought together the white managers and foremen of an automobile manufacturing plant with Black workers. Walter Kluvan, a white TV actor who had experience with Moreno's psychodrama techniques, and Dr. Denis Jackson, a Black psychiatrist, oversaw the discussion.[47] The film's title plays on a crucial issue exposed within their interactions: The white foremen refer to any Black man as "boy," an insult to their masculinity; but by the end of the film, the foremen have switched their references to "fella" and "man." The title also frames the open communication about their emotions that they undertake as a sign of maturity, recuperating open discussion of feelings from its femininized status.

In *Psychiatric Services*, a reviewer of the film argued that "teaching white foremen to be tolerant and teaching black workers to have proper work attitudes is a dead end: the only realistic solution is a program that will enhance two-way communication, rapport, mutual understanding, and respect."[48] Perhaps not surprisingly, *Psychiatric Services* reads the documentary in relation to how to maintain labor hierarchies. And while the film invites this reading, it is hard not to perceive the deeply racialized class issues in the two groups' interactions. Also, at no point is the fact that the Black workers will never be able to move up to foremen or managerial positions addressed, even though early scenes of job training show Black people presumably undergoing a job training program and working with typewriters and punch-card machines. They are, to be clear, probably being trained as typists and punch-card operators, not the loftiest of jobs. Nevertheless, these are the tools of the informatics industries, not the industrial Fordist economy: They are the tools of immaterial labor, not of autoworkers; they are the tools of a shift from industrial to informatics production that was roiling unionization efforts by Black workers in Detroit and elsewhere. The cultural and social context of the time suggests that its corporate sponsors expected the documentary would support an underlying anti-union, pro-capital logic. And in his own explanations of the making of the film, Greaves states his interest with the project stemmed from the dramatic possibilities of two people in conflict, unable to communicate.

Even with this setup of a liberal position of a therapeutic resolution to class and racialized conflict, the film nevertheless intervenes in discourses of Black male pathology by countering that with a portrait of *white men* as the problem.[49] Throughout the film, the Black participants are vocal, expressive, eager to talk and engage; one in particular, whose testimony concerns how a white foreman degraded him by parading him through the entire plant, is poetic in his delivery. The white participants, on the other hand, are reluctant, hesitant, quiet in their mode of speech. In fact, in one key scene it becomes clear that a white foreman's discomfort with the role-play—his inability to role-play as his Black employee—may spring from never imagining any position other than his own, and that the Black men's ease with role-play derives from their double consciousness. With the white actor and psychodramatist Walter Kluvan modeling for the white men an eager and expressive mode of white participation, and with their inability to match him, their participation style can be read as itself a failure to participate, an inability to meet the terms of the psychodrama at which the Black workers are so capable. Thus even though Lasch-Quinn's argument that sensitivity training contributed to the fall of the Civil Rights Movement is convincing, as an instance of racial sensitivity training this film suggests that *its mediation* provided its filmmaker a method to diminish the *discourse* of Black male pathology by recording and exhibiting the "pathology" of white emotional and communicative failure and the perhaps creative outcomes of Black double consciousness.

This instance of "encounter television" is distinct from *Black Ghetto Family*, which did not use psychodrama's techniques of role-switching and structured reenactments. Nevertheless, as concurrent uses of simulation to achieve similar goals—teaching white professionals, and a professional audience, better skills for interacting with working-class Black people—they merit comparison. In that both were audiovisually recorded, they evidence intersections among simulation, media, and racial liberalism in this period. When simulations, role-playing, and psychodrama were mobilized for "race relations" discourse, they joined racial liberalist goals of making white people sympathetic to Black Americans' experience, and at the same time conveyed, even if it was not their intent, that racial capitalism produced a racialized class struggle that simulation could only work to contain.

The Intersectional Critique of Simulation:
Waking Up from Media-Technological Dreams

A surprising instance of simulation with videotaped therapy appears in the Third World Newsreel film *A Dream Is What You Wake Up From* (1978). (By 1978, Newsreel, discussed in chapter 2, had evolved into Third World Newsreel.[50]) Made by Black filmmakers Larry Bullard and Carolyn Y. Johnson, members of Newsreel, the film has been described as "offering an experimental point of view of the african american class clash—working class vs. middle class" and as suggesting "that the ongoing traumas and derangements in the relations between men and women in black American families are a bitter legacy of the sexual and emotional traumas of slavery and Jim Crow."[51] The film includes a metafilmic moment of a videotaped counseling session, a film within a film that, as Pearl Bowser puts it, "imposes a distance between the audience and the exploding tensions to allow the viewer another perspective of the families within the film."[52] As I will argue, because this metafilmic moment depicts therapy, the film produces a critical spectatorial position toward psychotherapeutic discourses and practices, including as they manifest within visual techniques of recording and playback. Moreover, as the film blends documentary with narrative features, the indexicality of the counseling session is punctured, suggesting a critical spectatorial position toward the mediation of blackness and therapy. I will argue that this puncture of techniques of suture by which documentary constitutes itself as a truth discourse forces to the surface the relations among psychiatry, the filmic, and simulative logics. It makes manifest that staging and videotaping Black families in therapy within a racist visual culture functions to pathologize the black family; situated within the context of the film's thematizing of class struggle, it positions therapy and videotapes of therapy as instruments of heteropatriarchal class rule.

By 1978, simulative practices had permeated what historian Alice O'Connor has named the "poverty knowledge" industries.[53] In New York, the Urban Institute's Micro Analysis of Transfers to Households (MATH) microsimulation model was at the center of debates over welfare and food stamps. While I do not contend that the debates occurring within city, state, and federal agencies around these microsimulation models' predictions directly influenced the film, that the community of impoverished Black people that constituted one half of the film's storyline was at the center of these debates reminds us that Black families were taken as the object of microsimulation modeling for the purpose of apportioning state benefits. Thus I read the film's mediation of simulation, and its questioning of simulation within state-funded spaces of care, as commenting, albeit indirectly, on the abstract deployment of data in simulation modeling that had a direct, material effect on the possibilities for Black life and care.

The film opens with a scene of two women, casually dressed in shorts and tank tops, seated at a small kitchen table—that seminal trope of Black feminist thought—talking about one woman's husband beating her.[54] It then cuts to a public event on "The Black Family" at the Countee Cullen Library in Harlem, where Black women discuss the position of the Black woman since the 1960s. Much of the discussion echoes what the Combahee River Collective (CRC) had laid out, one year earlier, in their statement: that women in the Black Power movement were told their position "was prone"; that imperialism requires that Black women remain at the bottom of a hierarchy of oppressions; and that imperialism has found a way to make strong Black women look weak.[55] (In fact, I will argue here that Michelle Materre's interpretation of the film as showing a "class clash" between the Black middle and working classes might be revised in light of the context of the CRC and other Black feminist thought, that it illuminated the contradictions among rights movements that Black feminists were engaged with and the CRC's intersectional analysis—their term was "interlocking"—of oppressions.) A cut from this public forum where Black women engage in political discussion back to the two women sitting in a kitchen creates resonances between the political discourse and the private discourse. This suggests that the minute details of family life voiced by the two women realize the abstract political critiques voice at the public forum in the minute details of family life that the two women discuss. The personal and the political are sutured together, and the viewer is encouraged to understand the abuse the working-class Black woman experiences through the prism of the politics articulated at the "The Black Family" event.

A montage of black-and-white photographs of Black families follows, as the band Sweet Honey in the Rock sings the repeated line "That is my dream." These photographs venture backward in time, starting with the 1960s, then perhaps the 1920s, and their ordering suggests the film is describing the history of the Black family. Live action scenes then show Black men and women, overseen by men with guns, toiling in a what is perhaps a tobacco field. Another group of Black men, women, and children look on at them but are waved away by the white men. We are looking at post–Civil War indentured workers, one assumes. They plan an escape; later, at night, chased by men and dogs, they may achieve their escape, or they may not; the sequence ends with two men making it into a boat and rowing away from the bank, during which a woman's voice speaks, incants, in a rhythm suggestive of poetry. She says,

> Necklace of tears, bracelet of blood,
> my people have been sold
> in the marketplace, on the auction block, in the cotton fields,
>   on the docks.
> And you and I
> have both accepted
> the dream of free love
> and store-bought struggle
> that this selling of ourselves
> offers as unrequited revolution's reward.
> As the sun begins to rise,
> its rays of light caress the tops of the trees
> and outline the buildings on an empty street.
> Someone is waiting.

The next scene cuts to a suburban street, then to a living room where two Black children open Christmas gifts (the girl receives a white Barbie doll, one of the film's two instances of dominant white beauty culture), and their parents join them, dressed in luxurious bathrobes. The poem suggests that this couple has compromised in their attainment of suburban middle-class life ("store-bought struggle") and that the sexual revolution (the "dream of free love") deflected the energies needed for social revolution. Resonating with the film's other evocations of "dreams" and poetry—Sweet Honey in the Rock's song version of Langston Hughes's "Dream Variations," with its chorus, alluding to Hughes's "Harlem," of "nothing lights a fire like a dream deferred"—the end of the poem suggests there might be a new day beyond this compromise, perhaps a new identity ("someone is waiting"). With its decidedly cinematographic description of the sun's rise (the focus on how light bounces, highlights, shadows), the poem's penultimate line suggests this film itself is one vehicle for transport to this new day and this new "someone."

The film's title also indicates that dreams are mirages to be emerged from, and so, in the succeeding scenes, which document the middle-class couple's success in achieving suburban life, the viewer is alert for fractures and moments of dissonance, indications that their American dream life is the "selling out" of the poem. While they seem happy in their relationship, in one interview it becomes clear that the wife, Barbara (we never learn the husband's name), is less than satisfied with their move to the suburbs, as she is far from her work in New York City and has no friends where they are. Her husband explains that, when a white worker was promoted over him, he left his Wall Street job to work independently as a financial counselor for Black clients, and this new career required their move away from the city. As the husband names the quality of Barbara that attracted him to her—sophistication—this praise is spoken over exterior shots of a makeup advertisement featuring two white models. Because the film has marked this family's distinction from the kitchen-table working-class women, his words are implicated in a form of colorism. In effect, his praise for her belittles the working-class women who do not have these qualities.

These scenes cut back to the two women talking at the kitchen table, and from there to the scene of the central couple, called Mr. and Mrs. Fenway, receiving counseling from a group of three counselors, two men and one woman. The couple hash out their core issue—the wife has brought the husband to get help for his physical abuse—as the counselors try to get each to agree to modify behavior. As things get heated, the wife implies that the husband forces her to have sex; the female counselor then asks her if she'd like to talk about something here, in a space of relative safety, that she hasn't been able to talk to her husband about. The scene cuts back to the two women in the kitchen, where the woman we assume to be Mrs. Fenway tells her friend that the counseling session didn't help.

The suture—from the counseling session, where Mrs. Fenway mentions rape, to the kitchen table, where the woman mentions rape—suggests these are the same woman. Yet dissonance between how the two women dress, style themselves, and speak introduces a bit of doubt. And while the interview scenes and the discussion scenes are staged as live documentary, the counselors' delivery is odd enough to make the viewer wonder whether it is bad counseling or, perhaps, bad acting. Later in the film, as seen in figure 4.1, we see the end of the counseling session again; a slow zoom out reveals that it is being broadcast on a TV screen, from a videotape player, and that a group of men, sitting in a room where they are surrounded by shelves holding film canisters, are discussing the counseling session in relation to their ideas about gender roles.

This video recording viewed by the men is a psychiatric screening, a moment in which the psychotherapeutic is recorded for later broadcast and viewing. As a metafilmic moment, it suggests possibilities for a critical examination of spectatorship wielded within psychiatric screenings. The men articulate a critical perspective on the counseling session; for example, one remarks that the counselors' attempt to get the husband to agree to a com-

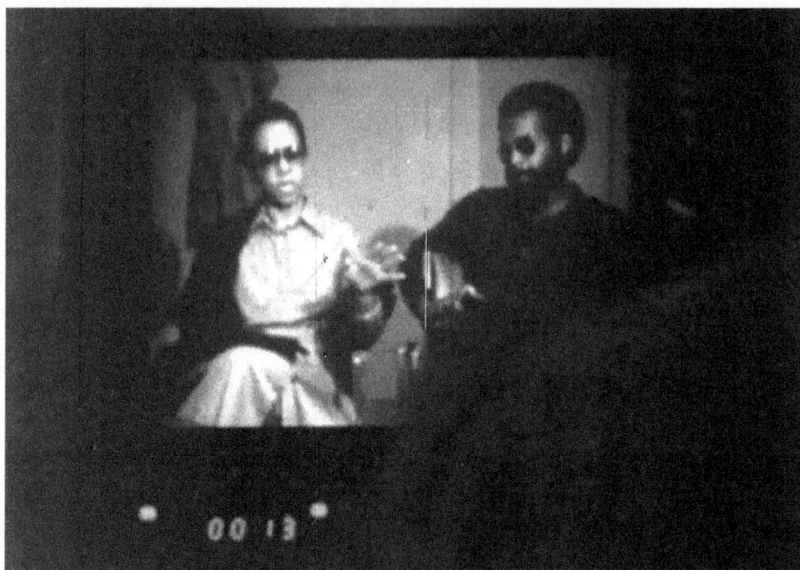

FIGURE 4.1. *A Dream Is What You Wake Up From* (1978).

promise will not result in the husband's deep understanding of the situation. As they talk among themselves, those men who articulate the deepest understanding of how cultural codes of masculinity have affected them do not refer to the videotape itself—in fact if anything, the videotape serves more as a launching point for discussion, as they quickly move from what is shown in the videotape to other topics. In this setting, the videotape indicates that a collective discussion is better equipped than an individual counseling session to address how the politics of gender, race, and class contribute to gendered forms of abuse. By showing the men engaged in a critical conversation about the counseling session, the procedures and discourses of counseling are opened up for critique through the act of Black spectatorship. As a film-within-a-film, this scene presses a critical examination of the film's spectatorial position as imbued with preconceptions of Black families; that is, in placing spectators in a position to consider whether the men's viewing responses are valid, spectators examine their own responses. One of the men articulates a sexist response, the kind of sexism the collective discussion shown at the film's beginning had outlined, and thus viewership itself is made available for critique: How is one's response to televisual and cinematic depictions of the Black family already determined by the sexism, heteropatriarchy, and racism that define the terms of that viewing?

In pressing the viewer to this critical engagement, the film discards the approach taken by the counselors—asking the man and woman to compromise—and sides with Mrs. Fenway's friend, who understands problems in Black heterosexual relationships to stem from economic oppression as it interlocks with structural racism as they interlock with sexism. I use the term "interlock" with specific reference to the CRC statement's use of it. One year before production of *A Dream Is What You Wake Up From*, the CRC authors wrote, "We are actively committed to struggling against racial, sexual, heterosexual, and class oppression, and see as our particular task the development of integrated analysis and practice based upon the fact that the major systems of oppression are interlocking."[56] Indeed, this is specifically the analysis offered by Mrs. Fenway's friend. For her, Mrs. Fenway's husband is subjected to racial and class oppression during his working day—"everything is going down the drain"—and when he comes home, "You're the only one he can rebel against, he can whup you, you ain't no sweat to him. So whatever they can do to him in society, we still get the end of the deal." Mrs. Fenway then describes a typical fight they have, where he comes home and complains that she hasn't made dinner, but she hasn't made dinner because there's no money for food. The film cuts to Barbara making dinner in her middle-class kitchen and talking about her optimistic outlook on life, drawing a stark contrast between the two women's economic status and how that status affects their capacities to fulfill expectations of gender roles in the heterosexual family.

The film concludes with a scene at the kitchen table, as the friend says, "The whole thing boils down to this: Do you think you can get him to come over to your side? . . . Do you think he can have you equal with him, not behind him. You know, 'Hey, let's lock arms, let's do this thing together.'" Notable is that the friend's suggestion hinges on a similar calculation employed by the counselors—equality means a form of equal compromise—and yet its underlying analytic, of interlocking oppressions, is entirely different. Her friend considers the repair of their relationship to be one component of a politics struggling against racial and class oppression. The counseling is critiqued as failing to instantiate a politics of the personal by replicating the patriarchal system that the film itself critiques.

Ultimately, like other works of independent Black filmmaking from this time, *A Dream Is What You Wake Up From* envisions Black families, and Black women, through narrative and formal modes that contest their envisioning in Hollywood filmmaking and emerging Black studio filmmaking. To evoke a phrase from LA Rebellion filmmakers, the film aims to "emancipate the image." Its refusal to conform to generic expectations—it uses the grammar of documentary even as an intertitle explains that parts of it are staged—formally realizes this image emancipation. *A Dream* deployed an experimental staged documentary style to realize Black feminist theory cinematically: in other words, to wrestle with how cinematic conventions "contained" the image that needed emancipating. A Third World Newsreel production and dedicated to Cuban radical filmmaker Sara Gomez and the Mozambique-born revolutionary worker Josina Machel, the film is limned by its gestures to third-world women's liberation struggles. It situates US Black women's lives within the interlocking oppressions of class, race, and gender, which also interlock with the imperialist project, referenced in tobacco farming, of resource extraction and extractive labor. It refutes cultural discourses of Black familial pathology and takes seriously Black women's individual and collective efforts toward liberation. Simulations and therapy are, in a sense, secondary to these primary concerns. Nevertheless, at the film's midpoint, this meta-filmic moment critiquing psychotherapy and its screen mediation, and the film's blurring of boundaries between narrative and documentary, between representation and the real, reveals psychotherapeutic mediations as pathologizing screens. The film illustrates that Black cultural production questioned the ontology of objectivity that had by 1978 attached to videotape, including the filmic objectivity that informed Greaves's experiment with psychodrama.

That a film engaged with Black feminist discourses would critique that ontology is not surprising. Black feminist work in this period assertively critiqued capitalist heteropatriarchy's delegitimizing of Black women's testimony. The film makes this critique in ways both diegetically explicit and formally implicit. It is explicit when a participant at the public forum states that "imperialism needs to make the strong woman look weak," and it is implicit when the men discussing the psychotherapeutic videotape discount the woman's motives. In the second instance, videotape cannot legitimate the Black woman's speech; instead, her testimony is recontained and delegitimized within heteropatriarchal visual culture codes that make her speech always suspect. Still, the men's discussion of the videotape moves them toward self-criticality, and, although they fail to receive the woman's testimony, they nevertheless model a self-critical gaze that hints, for the film's viewers, at the possibilities that inhere in critically engaging with audiovisual media. In this, the film presages bell hooks's oppositional gaze: It positions its black women viewers as wielders of modes of looking that might, as Sweet Honey in the Rock's lyrics put it, "light a fire."

Conclusion

With Macy Foundation funding, standardized patients became routine in medical training and assessment, and in 1993 the Association of American Medical Colleges certified them as a legitimate method for licensing exams. Researchers then began to develop standardized (simulated) patients to teach "interpersonal skills" and diagnostics. Today such research continues, including through computer-simulated and virtual reality patients, in educational contexts that stress principles such as "cultural competency" and diversity, equity, and inclusion (DEI). Or, as a 2021 review of virtual standardized patients (VSPs) in psychiatric and mental health professions training puts it, "Medical schools have perhaps never been more focused on training medical students and residents with a focus on diversity, equity, and inclusion."[57] The authors suggest that "VSPs could offer a range of skill development opportunities and experiential learning scenarios to improve DEI trainings relevant to treatment planning, case formulation, and communication among patients who are Black, Indigenous, or people of color. Similarly, the future establishment of VSP programs that support a standardized and validated evaluation of professional expertise and clinical skills may help address the risk of implicit bias among human raters. Such applications may be of particular value in geographic regions of the country where there exists an inadequate number of human standardized patients from underrepresented communities."[58] Here, the technology of simulation again serves as an instrument to overcome histories of discrimination and bias in mental health care, and it is again framed through a normative perspective that Others Black, Indigenous, or people of color. The culture of psychiatry distinguishes itself from those it has historically pathologized through its benevolent and Othering language, even as it promises to wield the new racial liberalism of DEI to provide "culturally competent" service. Simulations—computerized, videotaped, or live—reproduce psychiatry's fantasy of objectivity and its tenuous authority, granting it the sheen of "evidence-based" expertise. They allow the psychotherapeutic professions to contain the spillover within racial liberalist formulations.

One recent example of psychiatric ways of screening occurred in the wake of 2020's worldwide protests against the police and for racial justice. In the summer of 2020 and into the next year, like so many other institutions (museums, universities, archives) and organizations, the professional associations of psychiatry and psychology, the American Psychiatry Association (APA) and the American Psychological Association, participated in the now de rigueur genre of task forces and apology statements. The APA's "Presidential Task Force to Address Structural Racism Through Psychiatry" included in its final report this brief, yet not insignificant, note: that the APA's Council on Quality Care's Committee on Mental Health Information Technology "will be exploring ways to use [i]nformation technology to address racial and socioeconomic disparities, including the potential use of clinical decision support algorithms to remove some of the subjectivity and bias that enters into diagnosis and treatment."[1] This contemporary example of technology as remedy for psychiatry is, granted, a minor note in a much longer itemizing of actions that the APA intended to take; yet shortly thereafter claims that emerging tech can address racial disparities in "care" and biased psy professionals gained traction.

Consider the recent debut of so-called generative artificial intelligence (AI) and forms of psychiatric screeening such as the Black Female Therapist AI chatbot. According to the company's CEO (also a psychiatrist), the Black Female Therapist was programmmed to respect cultural differences and therefore could provide so-called culturally sensitive "care" for those Black people seeking help—while its host platform, ChatGPT, gobbles up sensitive information and data for whatever third-party uses it pleases.[2] Defending AI chatbots against that evergreen "garbage in, garbage out" criticism, one psychiatrist countered that an AI chatbot programmed by a Black mental health professional, or someone who worked in transgender care, might overcome some of the long-standing issues with reproducing bias that bedevil AI and its training data. Thus technological innovation again poses as a means to address psychiatry's failures through provisions of care that both its critics and its promoters acknowledge as subpar to other forms of therapy. Within today's highly networked data streams, however, when LexisNexis scores people's risk categories via their data profiles and when law enforcement can subpoena tech firms for archived data, it is worse than subpar: it is predatory inclusion.[3] It is racial capitalism masquerading as care.

Perhaps, instead of getting by with this latest iteration of a predatory psy-tech complex, you have found, or been found by, mutual aid networks that provide collective methods of care and work toward anticarceral futures. It is in light of our contemporary efforts to build anticarceral systems of care that this book has followed the slight shimmers of submerged moments when media and technologies of psychiatric control were contested and used to other ends. That its assembled archive ends with the 1970s reflects nothing more than the author's life exigencies and, perhaps, a sense that its chapters have adequately begun a project that others might continue. It is to join with the ongoing, developing crip theoretical critiques of our present, and out of love for the thrill seekers in the streets, that this book has constructed a minor, perhaps illuminating, genealogy of crip screens that counter psychiatry.

Acknowledgments

This book developed over many years with the support of archivists at the following institutions: University of California at Berkeley's Bancroft Library, Prelinger Archive, National Library of Medicine, Schomburg Center for Research in Black Culture, New York University Film Library, Columbia University Libraries, Paley Center for Media, Archives of the Albert Einstein College of Medicine, Wisconsin Historical Society, New York Public Library, American Association for University Women, and Library of Congress. I especially thank Sarah Eilers at the National Library of Medicine History of Medicine Division for fielding many requests between 2020 and 2022; her timely responses and the work she put into making films available electronically were crucial. This book is also indebted to Oren Jacoby and Sylvia Walton. I thank Jacoby profusely for taking the time to speak with me and for sharing with me some of the films discussed in chapter 3.

The close readings and broader claims of the book were strengthened through discussions with my former University of Texas (UT) at Dallas colleagues and with colleagues at other institutions. They also benefited from attendees of presentations at the University of California, Los Angeles; the University of California, Santa Barbara; Penn State University; Princeton University; the Society for Cinema and Media Studies; and UT Dallas's Feminist Research Collective, and from comments by anonymous reviewers for the *Journal of Cinema and Media Studies*, *Disability Studies Quarterly*, and Duke University Press. The writing of the book was supported by a University of Texas System Special Faculty Assignment, a sabbatical taken in 2020–21.

Liz Ault has been a magnanimous editor, supporting the project through all its stages and understanding my crip time signatures. I also thank Craig Willse, whose keen editorial work helped ensure that this project came together into what is hopefully a coherent whole. Thanks also to Bird Williams at Duke for thoughtful editing and production guidance.

To my crew—Moby, Stevie, Freddy, Ziggy, Tessa, Wolfie; Jen, Rebecca, Eman, Kim, Lisa, Josef, Sarah, Wendy, Hong-An—mad respect for all of you thrillseekers.

Notes

INTRODUCTION

Epigraph: Sanchez, "A Poem for Ella Fitzgerald" (1998).

1 Cohen, "Digital Devices."

2 In *Discriminating Data*, Wendy Chun discusses developments that built on Moreno's research, including Paul Lazarsfeld's 1950s study on friendship patterns, as well as other early eugenicists' developments of mathematical and computational logics that permeate technology today.

3 See, e.g., Hicks, *Talk with You Like a Woman*.

4 Morse, "The Farm as a Factor in Training Delinquent Girls."

5 Moreno, *Who Shall Survive?*, 3.

6 For an in-depth analysis of Moreno's eugenic philosophies and their relation to the creation of informatic value, see Franklin, *The Digitally Disposed*.

7 Stella is an instance of blackness both hypervisible and invisible, as per Browne, *The Surveillance of Blackness*.

8 Somerville, *Queering the Color Line*.

9 Spillers, "Mama's Baby, Papa's Maybe."

10 Moreno's revised 1953 edition, retitled *Who Shall Survive? Foundations of Sociometry, Group Psychotherapy and Sociodrama*, began with a one-hundred-page synopsis of his career leading up to the Hudson Prison research and extending past it, including detailing what Moreno saw as its ever-expanding influence on intellectual movements, clinical practices, and government policymaking. The applause would reach its fever pitch in the title of his autobiography, *Autobiography of a Genius*.

11 See, among others, Leys, *The Ascent of Affect*; Crawford, *The Atlas of AI*; Ekman, *Nonverbal Messages*.

12 In other work, Ekman made distinctions about his work as a "filmmaker" (i.e., his recorded interviews of depressed patients), a "film analyzer" (developing automated methods for VID-R), and as a "secondary investigator" (of films by Bateson, Mead, and other anthropologists). Unfortunately, this still does not clarify which recordings he used in developing his VID-R. Ekman, "Comment."

13 Although he would quickly turn to his more famous photograph analysis, there is a connection between this VID-R work within that turn: Both were funded under Defense Advanced Research Projects Agency grants; and, in a 1967 response to an article by social scientist Richard Sorenson about how to produce research films, Ekman promoted his videotape-computer system as parallel to, yet more efficient for retrieval purposes than Sorenson's suggestion of splicing titles into research

films. Also, in 1967, buoyed by the desire to "prove the cultural relativists wrong" (by which he meant Margaret Mead, who had attacked Ekman's work), Ekman traveled to Sorenson's research site in New Guinea, there taking photos and recording film to begin validating his universal human facial expressions project.

14 Ekman, *Nonverbal Messages*, 94. See also Ekman and Friesen, "A Tool for the Analysis of Motion Picture Film or Video Tape," 240; and Ekman, Friesen, and Taussig, "VID-R and SCAN."

15 Chun, "Queerying Homophily"; McPherson, "US Operating Systems"; Black, *IBM and the Holocaust*.

16 On science in captivity, see Visperas, *Skin Theory*; and Benjamin, *Captivating Technology*.

17 Beller, *The World Computer*.

18 See, e.g., Lea, *Digitizing Diagnosis*; Greene, *The Doctor Who Wasn't There*; and Zeavin, *The Distance Cure*.

19 Schalk and Kim, "Integrating Race," 35.

20 Schalk and Kim, "Integrating Race," 43.

21 On madness and its strategic inhabitations, see Bruce, *How to Go Mad Without Losing Your Mind*.

22 See, e.g., Gabbard and Gabbard, *Psychiatry*; Walker, *Couching Resistance*; DeAngelis, *Rx Hollywood*.

23 Muñoz, *Disidentifications*.

24 Obituary in *Down Beat*, cited in Nicholson, *Ella Fitzgerald*, 246n2.

25 Korall, *Drummin' Men*.

26 Wells, "Go Harlem"; Wells, "'A Dreadful Bit of Silliness.'"

27 Rosetta Reitz Papers, "Ella Fitzgerald," box 12, c. 1; Brooks, *Liner Notes for the Revolution*. Reitz composed some of her notes about Fitzgerald on a medication pad for high blood pressure—a mediated reminder of crip worldmaking through cultural preservation.

28 Sanchez, "A Poem for Ella Fitzgerald."

29 White et al., *Playing the Numbers*, 105; see also Harris, *Sex Workers, Psychics, and Number Runners*.

30 Nina Bernstein, "Ward of the State: The Gap in Ella Fitzgerald's Life," *New York Times*, June 23, 1996.

1. PSYCHIATRIC WAYS OF SCREENING IN THE LONG 1960S

1 Glueck, "Automation and Social Change."

2 Strobel et al., "Designing Psychiatric Computer Information Systems."

3 As Jackie Orr has argued through the example of Glueck's peers, Nathan Klein and Manfred Clynes, an informatics of biopsychiatry was envisioned as necessary for "governing mentalities" and instituting centralized command-and-control systems over potentially unruly populations. See Orr, "Biopsychiatry."

4 On the mid-1960s Senate hearings about the MMPI and constitutional rights, see Buchanan, "On Not 'Giving Psychology Away.'"

5   See Womack, *The Matter of Black Living.*

6   I draw here on work about cultural production as site of contestation, such as Brady, *Scales of Captivity,* and Womack, *The Matter of Black Living.*

7   Jefferson, *Digitize and Punish*; Bowker and Starr, *Sorting Things Out*; McIlwain, *Black Software.*

8   McIlwain, *Black Software.*

9   See, e.g., Hedlund, "Computers in Mental Health."

10 Hedlund, "Computers in Mental Health."

11 David Jardini analyzes the jockeying within various federal administrative units in the early 1960s to argue that the social welfare programs instituted under Great Society Initiatives, and in particular their emphasis on including the impoverished within decision-making and planning, worried high-ranking influential officials such as Robert McNamara. With years at the Department of Defense, characterized by a hierarchical structure and technical deployment of centralized systems analysis work for these officials, the decentralization and democratic structure of the initial social welfare programs did not deserve support, and their reluctance led them to insist that policy be backed by research and evaluative studies. "This fixation on policy research and evaluation accompanied systems analysis and program budgeting as these methods diffused from the Pentagon to the federal social welfare agencies." See Jardini, "Out of the Blue Yonder." See also Jefferson, *Digitize and Punish,* 41.

12 Brown, "Learning to Love Computers."

13 The full list of institutions is Texas Medical Center (Houston), Children's Hospital (Akron, OH), Johns Hopkins University School of Medicine (Baltimore, MD), the Institute of Living (Hartford, CT), Harvard Medical School (Cambridge, MA), Yale University Library (New Haven, CT), Wilmington Medical Center (Wilmington, NC), Tulane University (New Orleans, LA), the University of Texas Medical Branch (Galveston), Roswell Park Memorial Institute (Buffalo, NY), the University of Missouri (Columbia), and UCLA.

14 This ordinariness is distinct from other styles in industrial management films, for example, the McGraw Hill management documentaries analyzed by Ramon Reichert, which popularized management techniques to high schools and other nonexpert audiences and imported noncinematic visualizations like the circuit diagram and pictograms to spice up very mundane content. Reichert, "Behaviorism, Animation, and Effective Cinema."

15 See, e.g., Hookway, "Cockpit."

16 See, e.g., Nash, "Compliance of Hospitals and Health Agencies"; Reynolds, "The Federal Government's Use of Title VI."

17 Byrd and Clayton, *An American Health Dilemma.*

18 See, e.g., Ostherr, *Medical Visions*; MacKenzie, "'Mental Prophylaxis'"; Druick, "Before Education, Good Food and Health."

19 Jacoby and Anderson, "Scenario for Psychiatry," 43.

20 Briggs, *Reproducing Empire,* 110.

21 On Puerto Rico as social laboratory for development efforts, see Briggs, *Reproducing Empire*; Lapp, "The Rise and Fall of Puerto Rico." The study for which the

film was produced was ultimately published as Hill, Stycos, and Back, *The Family and Population Control*. In their research, these US social scientists showed the film along with a pamphlet about family planning in an effort to determine which one—print materials or audiovisual materials—was most effective as a persuasive device. The film's narration was in English, not Spanish.

22 Irving Lerner, the director, specialized in film noir, including *Murder by Contract* (1958) and *City of Fear* (1960).

23 "Council Offers Film Showing," *The Morning Record* (Meriden, CT), October 7, 1968; broadcast on local Sunday television, Channel 22 (Scranton, PA), "Television Program Logs for Entire Week," *The Scrantonian*, May 4, 1968, p. 8B; "'Bold New Approach' Film on Mental Health Feature of Church Dinner Tomorrow," *Glens Falls Times* (Glens Falls, NY), March 19, 1968, p. 10; "Tales of the Town," *The Billings* (MT) *Gazette*, November 10, 1967, p. 11; J. G. B., "Coming Through Your Front Door."

24 Felix, "The Community Mental Health Center," 162.

25 See W. Kaplan, *California Design*.

26 Spigel, *TV by Design*.

27 Spigel, *TV by Design*, 71.

28 See Menne, "Hitchcock's Closed Systems."

29 See, e.g., Siegert, *Cultural Techniques*.

30 Knoblauch, *The Architecture of Good Behavior*, 6.

31 Binkley, *Getting Loose*.

32 Binkley, *Getting Loose*.

33 See "Description Adapted from Documents in the NET Microfiche," https://americanarchive.org/catalog/cpb-aacip-75–44pk0t5j.

34 The full list is Horizon House; Spruce House; the Jefferson Mental Health/Retardation Center in Philadelphia; Fountain House in New York City; Wellmet in Boston; Willow House, a VA hospital in Menlo Park, California; and the Singer Zone Center in Rockford, Illinois.

35 For a detailed account of the film's production and subsequent litigation, see Benson and Anderson, *Reality Fictions*, chap. 2. The state's censorship of an audiovisual exposé of the inhumanity of mental institutions reminds us what was at stake in the visual culture of madness: biopower. Indeed, Wiseman's censored film became a political instrument as various Boston politicians, jockeying within their state's backlash to Great Society Initiatives, launched investigations of the conditions at Bridgewater—a hospital for the "criminally insane"—and wrested control of the prison from the Department of Corrections to reassign it to the Department of Mental Health.

36 In this moment of publicity around an exposé that featured a category called "the criminally insane," the series that I will analyze has to be considered as part of a broader cultural effort to distinguish among categories of "insanity": in effect, to capacitate some categories as rehabilitatable, and to continue debilitating other categories by marking them as unrehabilitatable. I argue that this was part of a broader social dynamic underway in this period that would eventually lead to the broad-

scale capacitation of those psychiatry could name "mentally ill," while those labeled "severely mentally ill" were consigned to zones of debilitation.

37   Orr, "Biopsychiatry and the Informatics of Diagnosis."

38   See Ekman, *Nonverbal Messages*.

39   See, e.g., Gates, *Our Biometric Future*; Benjamin, *Race After Technology*.

40   Wilmer published about his San Quentin work in "Television: Technical and Artistic Aspects of Videotape in Psychiatric Teaching." Video from that project is protected material, unviewable, in his archives at the Briscoe Center for American History, The University of Texas at Austin.

41   DeAngelis, *Rx Hollywood*.

42   See Ouellette, *Viewers Like You*. Ouellette argues that, with its mandate to provide "quality fare," as it was being defined by the highly educated, white bourgeois taste cultures of elite experts who bemoaned, to quote Newton Minow's infamous trashing of television, "the vast wasteland of television," public TV broadcast both such high Orientalist, patriarchal dramas as *The Galsworthy Saga* alongside such innovative, but ultimately discontinued, shows such as the Black soap opera *Bird of the Iron Feather*. At the same time, the film was produced through San Francisco's public affiliate, KQED, which, as Ouellette also notes, by 1972 had been identified by *TV Guide* as a station whose productions, which were often specifically antibusiness, pushed the envelope. (The station itself, according to Ouellette, performed internal research that found its audience perceived it as "radical" and "psychedelic" instead of "dull" and "educational.") This suggests that Wilmer's film provided the station with programming that continued to provide "quality fare" that also lent itself to the "psychedelic" nature of the station.

43   Television historian Lynn Spigel has shown that the credits of Alcoa Premier encapsulates television's trend, in this era, of incorporating the latest in graphic design, in this case "offer[ing] an aura of modern cosmopolitanism, bestowing the Alcoa Aluminum Corporation of America with a sense of progress through design" ("Back to the Drawing Board," 36). Although "People Need People" is outside my focus here, it is interesting to note that the first episode of a series itself permeated with notions of progress through design concerned an experiment in new forms of psychiatric ward living.

44   Wilmer, "Innovative Uses of Videotape"; Wilmer, "Television: Technical and Artistic," 1967; Wilmer, "Television as Participant Recorder."

45   Grimaldi, "Televising Psyche."

46   Wilmer, "Feedback," 11.

47   Kane, "The Tragedy of Radical Subjectivity"; Grimaldi, "Televising Psyche."

48   For more on these experiments, see, e.g., Rossi-Snook and Tilton, "'Don't Be a Segregationist'"; and Griffis, "Teenage Moviemaking on the Lower East Side."

49   Halleck, *Hand-Held Visions*; Gordon-Burroughs, "Looking Back and Away"; Weinstein, *The Pathological Family*.

50   Chalfen and Haley, "Reaction," 91.

51   Chalfen and Haley, "Reaction," 92.

52   Chalfen and Haley, "Reaction," 92.

53 Chalfen and Haley, "Reaction," 95.

54 Weinstein, *The Pathological Family*, 170.

55 A later article documented the investigators' broader participatory media research project, in which they gathered data to compare white, Black, girls', and boys' filmmaking. See Chalfen, "A Sociovidistic Approach to Children's Filmmaking."

56 Metzl, *The Protest Psychosis*.

57 Hardison, "Theorizing Jane Crow," 56.

58 Benjamin, "Informed Refusal."

59 Womack, *The Matter of Black Living*.

60 Bruce, *How to Go Mad Without Losing Your Mind*.

2. FEMINIST-OF-COLOR ACTIVISM AND INFORMATION JUSTICE AT LINCOLN HOSPITAL

1 See, e.g., Soares, "Joy, Rage, and Activism"; Fernández, *The Young Lords*; Nelson, *Women of Color and the Reproductive Rights Movement*; and Morales, *Through the Eyes of Rebel Women*.

2 McKinney, *Information Activism*.

3 Schalk and Kim, "Integrating Race."

4 The two films were *Uptown*, the one discussed here, and *Storefront* (dir. Herbert Danska; 1967). One review of *Storefront* indicates that it provided a 49-minute in-depth account of the training of community workers (Neher, "Review of *Storefront*"). The 1967 screening of *Storefront* at PS 150 in the South Bronx was attended by New York City's mayor and the Bronx borough president. See "Movie Premiered in Ghetto Area," press release, October 30, 1967, Albert Einstein College of Medicine Archives. I have not been able to recover any copies of *Storefront*.

5 Danska is best known today for his independent 1970 film *Right On!* about the Last Poets, a Harlem group.

6 Another productive comparison for this documentary would be CBS's prime-time *East Side/West Side* (1963–64), which also featured a social worker (played by George C. Scott) working in a multiethnic urban community. Aniko Bodroghkozy argues that episodes that focus "on race issues brought to maximum discursive visibility a cultural preoccupation with the place of African Americans in American society and the appropriate response by white liberals" (Bodroghkozy, *Equal Time*, 157). While *East Side/West Side* was entertainment, not a documentary, I argue here that *Manhattan Battleground* similarly addressed itself to white liberals.

7 See also Jade Davis on this era's turn to empathy culture in *The Other Side of Empathy*.

8 This mirrors the nonconventional sensibility evident in Danska's other work. The promotional posters for *Right On!* described it as "a conspiracy of ritual, street theater, soul music and cinema," formally mimicking poetry by emphasizing sound over visuals.

9 Peck and Struening, "A Community Mental Health Program," 195.

10 Peck and Struening, "A Community Mental Health Program," 197.

11 Neher, "Review of *Uptown*," 218-a.

12 On emerging studies that intervene in computing as white male, see, e.g., Rankin, *A People's History*; on informational labor within lesbian activism, see McKinney, *Information Activism*.

13 *New Architecture for Mental Health*, 22.

14 Fernández, *The Young Lords*, 275.

15 Mullan, *White Coat, Clenched Fist*.

16 Lehman, Struening, and Darling, "Lincoln Hospital," 102.

17 Lehman, Struening, and Darling, "Lincoln Hospital," 104.

18 Lehman, Struening, and Darling, "Lincoln Hospital," 104.

19 From what I have been able to ascertain, the programming staff were paid four times the monthly salary of nonprofessional staff. See Lehman, Struening, and Darling, "Lincoln Hospital," 110.

20 Peck and Struening, "A Community Mental Health Program," 205.

21 Collins, "Evaluative Research in Community Psychiatry," 99–100.

22 Peck and Struening, "A Community Mental Health Program," 205.

23 Lehman, Struening, and Darling, "Lincoln Hospital," 101–11.

24 Struening, Rabkin, and Peck, "Migration and Ethnic Membership."

25 Ehrenreich and Ehrenreich, *The American Health Empire*, 256; Kaplan and Roman, *The Organization and Delivery of Mental Health Services*.

26 Peck and Struening, "A Community Mental Health Program," 193.

27 Fernández, *The Young Lords*.

28 Mullan, *White Coat, Clenched Fist*, 147.

29 Mullan, *White Coat, Clenched Fist*, 148.

30 Lincoln Collective Newsletter, n.d. (est. 1971), Fitzhugh Mullan Papers, box 2, folder 5, Wisconsin Historical Society.

31 Lincoln Collective Newsletter, n.d. (est. 1971), Fitzhugh Mullan Papers, box 2, folder 5, Wisconsin Historical Society.

32 Lincoln Hospital, Department of Pediatrics, Education Committee Report, n.d., Fitzhugh Mullan Papers, box 2, folder 5, Wisconsin Historical Society.

33 Rodriguez-Trías, "The Hospital as a Community Facility," 1423.

34 William Bronston Papers, carton 3, folder 33, Special Collections, Bancroft Library, University of California at Berkeley.

35 See, e.g., Fernández, *The Young Lords*, 298–99.

36 Fernández, *The Young Lords*; Young, *Soul Power*.

37 See, e.g., Young, *Soul Power*; Adamson, *Enduring Images*; Robé, "Detroit Rising"; Nichols, *Newsreel*; Renov, "Newsreel."

38 Young, *Soul Power*, 100–144.

39 Young, *Soul Power*.

An earlier version of this chapter appeared as Banner, "Mental Health vs. Mutual Aid."

1 Schalk, "The Black Disability Politics."
2 Kim, "Toward a Crip-of-Color Critique."
3 McRuer, "In Focus"; Field and Gordon, *Screening Race*.
4 On the media industries, Black film crews, and Harlem in particular, see Griffis, "'Open the Door.'"
5 Ostherr, *Medical Visions*, 81.
6 The film can be viewed at https://www.youtube.com/watch?v=rH6K3Lm2wZ4 and https://catalog.archives.gov/id/88815.
7 Cartwright, *Screening the Body*.
8 Ostherr, *Medical Visions*.
9 See, in particular, Parascandola, "Syphilis at the Cinema."
10 Markowitz and Rosner, *Children, Race, and Power*, chap. 6, "Juvenile Delinquency and the Politics of Community Action."
11 It is entirely possible that Jacoby also wanted Black crew due to ongoing racial tensions in New York that were affecting film productions. However, there is no explicit evidence for this in the existing production notes. See Griffis, "'Open the Door.'"
12 Portions of the script are located in the Mayfield Papers at the Schomburg Center for Research into Black Culture, New York.
13 Moynihan, *The Negro Family*.
14 Mumford, "Untangling Pathology."
15 Bloom and Martin, *Black Against Empire*.
16 "NCCD Film, Irving Jacoby Producer," Gerald Markowitz and David Rosner Papers, Rare Book and Manuscript Library. Columbia University, New York.
17 "The Mental Health Film Board Announces the Release of Irving Jacoby's Hitch," n.d.; "NCCD Film, Irving Jacoby Producer," both in Markowitz and Rosner Papers.
18 Letter from Samuel Walton, director of We Care, to Linda Gillies, director of the Astor Foundation, "First Draft Proposal," October 6, 1976, Vincent Astor Foundation Records, Grant Files, 1976, We Care, New York Public Library Manuscripts, Archives, and Rare Books Division, New York.
19 Markowitz and Rosner, *Children, Race, and Power*, 208–13.
20 "We Care Group, 1969–1973," Ella Baker Papers, box 13, folder 36, Schomburg Center; letter from Ana Maria Stephens, director of community relations for ABC, to Sam Walton, November 21, 1973, box 3, file 19, "NCCD—We Care Group General," Markowitz and Rosner Papers.
21 French had at this point appeared as a character in an episode of *The Bill Cosby Show*.
22 The National Memorial African Bookstore was established in 1933 by Lewis Michaux, a Garveyite. Malcolm X gravitated to the bookstore and bookseller, giving speeches outside the store by 1964. See Emblidge, "Rallying Point."

23 I deliberately use the nonstigmatizing formulation "person experiencing addiction" rather than the stigmatizing (by essentializing) formulation "the addict."

24 It is difficult to ascertain whether the sound-level disjuncture happened diegetically or in postproduction. In either case, it was not leveled out in postproduction, indicating its intentional use.

25 In *Making a Promised Land*, Paula Massood describes how Harlem had come to be represented through the sociological gaze, first through the photo-text genre, and then in independent films such as *The Quiet One*, which combined documentary and fiction.

26 Massood, *Black City Cinema*, 85. Massood discusses flâneur moments in Blaxploitation films, where the main character walks through city streets and leads viewers on a tour.

27 Markowitz and Rosner, *Children, Race, and Power*, 212, drawing from Mitchell and Snyder's influential *Narrative Prosthesis*.

28 Schalk, "Black Disability Gone Viral."

29 Ferguson, *Aberrations in Black*.

30 Chen et al., *Crip Genealogies*.

31 Kim, "Toward a Crip-of-Color Critique," drawing on Gilmore, 2009.

32 O'Connor, *Poverty Knowledge*, chap. 9.

4. COUNTERING PSYCHIATRIC WAYS OF SIMULATING/RACIALIZING PATIENTS

Epigraph: Cleaver, *Soul on Ice* (1968), 11.

1 E.g., Wald, *Crossing the Line*.

2 Gaines, *Black for a Day*, 66.

3 Lasch-Quinn, *Race Experts*.

4 Edwards, *The Closed World*.

5 Raser, *Simulation and Society*.

6 Inbar and Stoll, *Simulation and Gaming in Social Science*.

7 Sprehe and Michielutte, "Simulation of Social Mobility."

8 Freeman and Sunshine, *Patterns of Residential Segregation*.

9 Wilson, "Review of GHETTO."

10 Light, *From Warfare to Welfare*.

11 O'Connor, *Poverty Knowledge*.

12 Murphy, *Rewriting Indie Cinema*, 7.

13 See Buchanan and Swink, "Golden Age of Psychodrama." On psychodrama, Saint Elizabeths, and racialization, see Summers, *Madness in the City of Magnificent Intentions*.

14 See Nolte, *Philosophy, Theory and Methods of J. L. Moreno*, 205–6; Hare and Hare, *J. L. Moreno*, 59–62.

15 Moreno himself noted the usefulness of portable video, recording, in 1964, his own work for subsequent closed-circuit TV exhibition at a mental hospital in California ("Psychodrama in Action").

16 Howard Barrows is generally considered to be the innovator of the standardized patient in medicine. What's interesting for the history I am tracing here is that, while most of Barrows's medical colleagues were reluctant to indulge in the "too-Hollywood" standardized patient, but the University of Southern California psychiatry unit went ahead with it and recorded videotapes of actors playing the role of psychiatric patients, which circulated within the department. See Barrows, "Simulated Patients in Medical Teaching," 676.
17 Delaney, "Simulation Techniques in Counselor Education," 183.
18 Claiborn and Lemberg, "A Simulated Mental Hospital"; Orlando, "The Mock Ward."
19 Bellman's report from RAND to the National Institutes of Health and his peer-reviewed publications occlude an important detail mentioned in his memoir, *Eye of the Hurricane*, where he notes that the 1973 book he published (Bellman and Smith, *Simulation in Human Systems*), a much broader summary of psychiatry and simulation, grew out of his interest in the work done by an assistant, Polly Kell, who worked at Resthaven, a "mental health institution" close to the University of Southern California in Chinatown. The center served, among others, local Nissei. In 1972, Resthaven was taken over by Asian American leftists, who demanded the center serve the community. In this context, "Dr. Strangelove" was a psycho-entific choice.
20 Bellman and Kurland, "On the Construction of a Simulation," iii.
21 Bellman and Kurland, "On the Construction of a Simulation," 4.
22 Bellman, Friend, and Kurland, "Simulation of the Initial Psychiatric Interview," 389.
23 Hayles, *How We Became Posthuman*; McPherson, "US Operating Systems." Bellman was certainly not the only programmer working at this time. Spurred by the example of a now-infamous simulated therapist, Weizenbaum's computer program ELIZA of 1964, computer researchers developed, in 1967, COMPUTEST, a computer program that could simulate both patient and therapist, with improvement of clinical skills again offered as the program's justification. See Starkweather, Kamp, and Monto, "Psychiatric Interview Simulation by Computer"; Weizenbaum, "ELIZA."
24 Bailey, "The Flexner Report"; Duffy, "The Flexner Report—100 Years Later."
25 Hummel, Lichtenberg, and Shaffer, "CLIENT 1," 164.
26 Lichtenberg, Hummel, and Shaffer, "CLIENT 1."
27 Underman, *Feeling Medicine*.
28 Bryson, "Training Counselors."
29 Colby, "Experimental Treatment of Neurotic Computer Programs," 220.
30 Corsini, *Role Playing in Psychotherapy*, ix.
31 Orr, *Panic Diaries*, 11.
32 Orr, *Panic Diaries*, 13.
33 Sager, Brayboy, and Waxenberg, *Black Ghetto Family*.
34 Sager, Brayboy, and Waxenberg, *Black Ghetto Family*, 221.
35 Doyle, *Psychiatry and Racial Liberalism*.

36 Cleaver, *Soul on Ice*, 30.

37 *Ritual Murder* (1978), a one-act play by Tony Dent, featured Thomas Brayboy as a main character.

38 Sager, Brayboy, and Waxenberg, *Black Ghetto Family*, 77.

39 Binkley, *Getting Loose*.

40 Weinstein, *The Pathological Family*.

41 Weinstein, *The Pathological Family*, 111.

42 Ackerman quoted in Weinstein, *The Pathological Family*, 146.

43 William Greaves, "100 Madison Avenues Will Be of No Help," *New York Times*, August 9, 1970, 81.

44 While Greaves's articulation of the aim of "encounter television" as therapy for an emotionally disturbed population, one that would decrease polarization, can be seen as a conservative move (in effect marking out as "extreme" the very legitimate political program of the Black Panthers, an early form of both-sides-ism), Greaves was also using psy rhetoric that would appeal to readers of the *New York Times* arts section. Additionally, by sweeping both white America and Black America into the category of pathological, Greaves eschewed the cultural discourse that assigned only Blackness to pathology. Nevertheless, as a Black media producer of rising influence in 1970, one suspects Greaves mobilized a discursive frame most palatable to the educated readership of the *New York Times*.

45 Greaves, "Log: In the Company of Men," 34.

46 Murphy, "The Documentary as Sociodrama."

47 Jackson was also the author of the Black militant novel *The Black Commandos*. In an interview, Jackson stated, "I am not interested in destroying white people . . . [b]ut in saving them. White people need to see that the sickness of racial prejudice which motivates them against the Negro is ultimately self-destructive and will only lead to disaster" (quoted in Peavy, "Pop Art and the Black Revolution," 212).

48 Neher, "Review of *In the Company of Men*," 31a–32.

49 Lasch-Quinn, *Race Experts*.

50 Young, *Soul Power*.

51 Materre, "Capture and Release," 152; Brody, "A Rare Film about Gendered Oppression."

52 Bowser, "Review," 89.

53 O'Connor, *Poverty Knowledge*.

54 Although the woman-of-color publisher Kitchen Table Press was not founded until two years later, Verna-Mae Grosvenor contributed "The Kitchen Crisis" to Toni Cade Bambara's widely read *The Black Woman* anthology of 1970.

55 Combahee River Collective, "Combahee River Collective Statement."

56 Combahee River Collective, "Combahee River Collective Statement," 362.

57 Reger et al., "Virtual Standardized Patients," 63.

58 Reger et al., "Virtual Standardized Patients," 62.

1   APA Task Force, "Final Report of the Presidential Task Force on Structural Racism Through Psychiatry, May 11, 2021," https://www.psychiatry.org/getmedia/bf561da0 -cd36-4e8e-9d65-17b12d7dd4a1/APA-Report-of-Task-Force-on-Structural-Racism -to-BOT-05112021.pdf.

2   L'Oréal Blackett, "I Spoke to Chat GPT's 'Black Female Therapist.' Will AI Save Our Mental Health?," *Refinery29*, March 13, 2024, https://www.refinery29.com/en-us /artificial-intelligence-chat-gpt-black-mental-health.

3   Taylor, *Race for Profit*.

Bibliography

ARCHIVES CONSULTED

Albert Einstein College of Medicine Archives
Ella Baker Papers, Schomburg Center for Research into Black Culture, New York
Fitzhugh Mullan Papers, Wisconsin Historical Society
Gerald Markowitz and David Rosner Papers, Columbia University
Harry Wilmer Papers, Briscoe Center for American History, The University of Texas at Austin
Julian Mayfield Papers, Schomburg Center for Research into Black Culture, New York
National Library of Medicine, History of Medicine, Films
Paley Center for Media, Los Angeles
Prelinger Library, San Francisco
Prison Public Memory Project, https://www.prisonpublicmemory.org
Rosetta Reitz Papers, David M. Rubenstein Rare Book & Manuscript Library, Duke University Library
Vincent Astor Foundation Records, Grant Files, 1976, We Care, New York Public Library Manuscripts, Archives, and Rare Books Division
William Bronston Papers, Bancroft Library, University of California, Berkeley

WORKS CITED

Adamson, Morgan. *Enduring Images: A Future History of New Left Cinema*. Minneapolis: University of Minnesota Press, 2018.
Bailey, Moya. "The Flexner Report: Standardizing Medical Students Through Region-, Gender-, and Race-Based Hierarchies." *American Journal of Law and Medicine* 43, nos. 2–3 (2017): 209–23.
Banner, Olivia. "Mental Health vs. Mutual Aid: Competing Visions of Care in Black-Authored Films in the 1970s." Special issue, Origins, Objects, Orientations: New Histories and Theories of Race and Disability, edited by Kelsey Henry, Anna Hinton, and Sony Coráñez Bolton. *Disability Studies Quarterly* 43, no. 1 (2023). https://dsq-sds.org/index.php/dsq/article/view/9681/8016.
Barrows, Howard. "Simulated Patients in Medical Teaching." *Canadian Medical Association Journal, Structural Stigma and Population Health* 98 (1968): 674–76.
Beller, Jonathan. *The World Computer: Derivative Conditions of Racial Capitalism*. Durham, NC: Duke University Press, 2021.

Bellman, Richard, Merril B. Friend, and Leonard Kurland. "Simulation of the Initial Psychiatric Interview." *Behavioral Science* 11, no. 5 (1966): 389–99.

Bellman, Richard, and Leonard Kurland. "On the Construction of a Simulation of the Initial Psychiatric Interview." Santa Monica, CA: RAND Corporation, 1964.

Bellman, Richard, and Charlene Smith. *Simulation in Human Systems: Decision-Making in Psychotherapy.* New York: John Wiley and Sons, 1973.

Benjamin, Ruha, ed. *Captivating Technology: Race, Carceral Technoscience, and Liberatory Imagination in Everyday Life.* Durham, NC: Duke University Press, 2019.

Benjamin, Ruha. "Informed Refusal: Toward a Justice-Based Bioethics." *Science, Technology, and Human Values* 41, no. 6 (2016): 967–90.

Benjamin, Ruha. *Race After Technology: Abolitionist Tools for the New Jim Code.* New York: Polity Press, 2019.

Benson, Thomas, and Carolyn Anderson. *Reality Fictions: The Films of Frederick Wiseman.* Carbondale: Southern Illinois University Press, 1989.

Berne, Erik. *Games People Play: The Psychology of Human Relationships.* New York: Grove Press, 1964.

Binkley, Sam. *Getting Loose: Lifestyle Consumption in the 1970s.* Durham, NC: Duke University Press, 2007.

Black, Edwin. *IBM and the Holocaust: The Strategic Alliance Between Nazi Germany and America's Most Powerful Corporation.* New York: Crown, 2001.

Bloom, Joshua, and Waldo E. Martin. *Black Against Empire: The History and Politics of the Black Panther Party.* Berkeley: University of California Press, 2016.

Bodroghkozy, Aniko. *Equal Time: Television and the Civil Rights Movement.* Urbana: University of Illinois Press, 2012.

Bowker, Geoffrey, and Susan Leigh Starr. *Sorting Things Out: Classification and Its Consequences.* Cambridge, MA: MIT Press, 1999.

Bowser, Pearl. "Review of *A Dream Is What You Wake Up From.*" *Black Scholar* (March–April 1980): 89–90.

Brady, Mary Pat. *Scales of Captivity: Racial Capitalism and the Latinx Child.* Durham, NC: Duke University Press, 2022.

Briggs, Laura. *Reproducing Empire: Race, Sex, Science, and US Imperialism in Puerto Rico.* Berkeley: University of California Press, 2003.

Brody, Richard. "A Rare Film About Gendered Oppression in African-American Family Life." *New Yorker*, May 15, 2018. https://www.newyorker.com/culture /richard-brody /a-rare-film-about-gendered-oppression-in-african-american-family-life.

Brooks, Daphne A. *Liner Notes for the Revolution: The Intellectual Life of Black Feminist Sound.* Cambridge, MA: Belknap Press, 2021.

Brown, Logan. "Learning to Love Computers: Useful Cinema and the Mediation of American Computing, 1958–62." *Technology and Culture* 63, no. 3 (2022): 655–88.

Browne, Simone. *Dark Matters: On the Surveillance of Blackness.* Durham, NC: Duke University Press, 2015.

Bruce, La Marr Jurelle. *How to Go Mad Without Losing Your Mind: Madness and Black Radical Creativity.* Durham, NC: Duke University Press, 2021.

Bruce, La Marr Jurelle. "Mad Is a Place; or, the Slave Ship Tows the Ship of Fools." *American Quarterly* 69, no. 2 (2017): 303–6.

Bryson, Seymour. "Training Counselors Through Simulated Racial Encounters." *Journal of Non-White Concerns in Personnel and Guidance* 2, no. 4 (1974): 218–23.

Buchanan, Dale Richard, and David Franklin Swink. "Golden Age of Psychodrama at Saint Elizabeths Hospital (1939–2004)." *Journal of Psychodrama, Sociometry, and Group Psychotherapy* 65, no. 1 (2017): 9–32.

Buchanan, Roderick. "On Not 'Giving Psychology Away': The Minnesota Multiphasic Personality Inventory and Public Controversy over Testing in the 1960s." *History of Psychology* 5, no. 3 (2002): 284–309.

Byrd, W. Michael, and Linda A. Clayton. *An American Health Dilemma: Race, Medicine, and Health Care in the United States 1900–2000*. New York: Routledge, 2001.

Cartwright, Lisa. *Screening the Body: Tracing Medicine's Visual Culture*. Minneapolis: University of Minnesota Press, 1995.

Chalfen, Richard. "A Sociovidistic Approach to Children's Filmmaking: The Philadelphia Project." *Studies in Visual Communication* 7, no. 1 (1981): 2–32.

Chalfen, Richard, and Jay Haley. "Reaction to Socio-Documentary Film Research in a Mental Health Clinic." *American Journal of Orthopsychiatry* 41, no. 1 (1971): 91–100.

Chen, Mel, Alison Kafer, Eunjung Kim, and Julie Avril Minich, eds. *Crip Genealogies*. Durham, NC: Duke University Press, 2023.

Chun, Wendy Hui Kyong. *Discriminating Data: Correlation, Neighborhoods, and the New Politics of Recognition*. Cambridge, MA: MIT Press, 2021.

Chun, Wendy Hui Kyong. "Queerying Homophily." In *Pattern Discrimination*, ed. Clemens Apprich, Wendy Hui Kyong Chun, Florian Cramer, and Hito Seyerl, 59–98. Minneapolis: University of Minnesota Press, 2018.

Claiborn, William L., and Raymond W. Lemberg. "A Simulated Mental Hospital as an Undergraduate Teaching Device." *Teaching of Psychology* 1, no. 1 (1974): 38–40.

Clarke, John Henrik, ed. *William Styron's Nat Turner: Ten Black Writers Respond*. Boston: Beacon Press, 1968.

Cleaver, Eldridge. *Soul on Ice*. New York: Delta Books, 1999. Originally published 1968.

Cohen, Sandy. "Digital Devices Could Reveal Clues About Mental Health." *UCLA News and Insights*, May 31, 2022. https://www.uclahealth.org/news/article/digital-devices -could-reveal-clues-about-mental-health.

Colby, Kenneth. "Experimental Treatment of Neurotic Computer Programs." *Archives of General Psychiatry* 10 (March 1964): 220.

Collins, Jerome A. "Evaluative Research in Community Psychiatry." *Psychiatric Services* 19, no. 4 (1968): 99–100.

Combahee River Collective. "Combahee River Collective Statement." In *Capitalist Patriarchy and the Case for Socialist Feminism*, ed. Zillah Eisenstein, 362–72. New York: Monthly Review Press, 1978.

Corsini, Raymond. *Role Playing in Psychotherapy*. New York: Routledge, 2017. Originally published 1966.

Crawford, Kate. *The Atlas of AI*. New Haven, CT: Yale University Press, 2021.

Davis, Jade. *The Other Side of Empathy*. Durham, NC: Duke University Press, 2023.

DeAngelis, Michael. *Rx Hollywood: Cinema and Therapy in the 1960s*. Albany, NY: SUNY Press, 2018.

Delaney, Daniel J. "Simulation Techniques in Counselor Education: Proposal of a Unique Approach." *Counselor Education and Supervision* 8, no. 3 (1969): 183.

Doyle, Dennis. *Psychiatry and Racial Liberalism in Harlem, 1936–1968*. Woodbridge, UK: Boydell and Brewer, 2016.

Duffy, Thomas P. "The Flexner Report—100 Years Later." *Yale Journal of Biology and Medicine* 84, no. 3 (2011): 269–76.

Edwards, Paul. *The Closed World: Computers and the Politics of Discourse in Cold War America*. Cambridge, MA: MIT Press, 1996.

Ehrenreich, Barbara, and John Ehrenreich. *The American Health Empire: Power, Profits, and Politics*. New York: Vintage, 1970.

Ekman, Paul. "'Comment' to E. Richard Sorenson, 'A Research Film Program in the Study of Changing Man.'" *Current Anthropology* 8, no. 5 (1967): 462–63.

Ekman, Paul. *Nonverbal Messages: Cracking the Code: My Life's Pursuit*. San Francisco: Paul Ekman Group, 2016.

Ekman, Paul, and Wallace V. Friesen. "A Tool for the Analysis of Motion Picture Film or Video Tape." *American Psychologist* 24, no. 3 (1969): 240–43.

Ekman, Paul, Wallace Friesen, and Thomas Taussig. "VID-R and SCAN: Tools and Methods for the Automated Analysis of Visual Records." In *The Analysis of Communication Content: Developments in Scientific Theories and Concepts*, edited by George Gerener et al., 297–313. New York: Robert E. Krieger, 1978.

Emblidge, David. "Rallying Point: Lewis Michaux's National Memorial African Bookstore." *Publishing Research Quarterly* 24, no. 4 (December 1, 2008): 267–76.

Erevelles, Nirmala. *Disability and Difference in Global Contexts: Enabling a Transformative Body Politic*. New York: Palgrave Macmillan, 2011.

Fanon, Frantz. *Black Skin, White Masks*. New York: Grove Press, 1967.

Felix, Robert. "The Community Mental Health Center, a New Concept." *Architectural Record* (November 1963): 162–64.

Ferguson, Roderick. *Aberrations in Black: Toward a Queer of Color Critique*. Minneapolis: University of Minnesota Press, 2004.

Fernández, Johanna. *The Young Lords: A Radical History*. Chapel Hill: University of North Carolina Press, 2019.

Field, Allyson Nadia, and Marsha Gordon, eds. *Screening Race in American Nontheatrical Film*. Durham, NC: Duke University Press, 2019.

Franklin, Seb. *The Digitally Disposed: Racial Capitalism and the Informatics of Value*. Minneapolis: University of Minnesota Press, 2021.

Freeman, Linton C., and Morris H. Sunshine. *Patterns of Residential Segregation*. Cambridge, MA: Schenkman Publishing, 1970.

Gabbard, Glen O., and Kris Gabbard. *Psychiatry and the Cinema*. Washington, DC: American Psychiatric Association, 1999.

Gaines, Alisha. *Black for a Day: White Fantasies of Race and Empathy*. Chapel Hill: University of North Carolina Press, 2017.

Gates, Kelly. *Our Biometric Future: Facial Recognition Technology and the Culture of Surveillance*. New York: NYU Press, 2011.

Gilmore, Ruthie. *Golden Gulag: Prisons, Surplus, Crisis, and Opposition in Globalizing California*. Berkeley: University of California Press, 2007.

Glueck, Jr., Bernard. "Automation and Social Change." *Comprehensive Psychiatry* 8, no. 6 (1967): 441–49.

Gordon-Burroughs, Jessica. "Looking Back and Away: Jaime Barrios's Film Club (1968)." *Discourse* 42, no. 3 (2020): 281–304.

Greaves, William. "Log: In the Company of Men." *Film Library Quarterly* 3, no. 1 (Winter 1969–70): 34.

Greene, Jeremy. *The Doctor Who Wasn't There: Technology, History, and the Limits of Telehealth*. Chicago: University of Chicago Press, 2022.

Griffin, John Howard. *Black Like Me*. Boston: Houghton Mifflin, 1961.

Griffis, Noelle. "'Open the Door and I'll Get It for Myself': Minority Production Assistant Programs and the Politics of the Urban Location Shoot, 1969–1974." *Journal of Cinema and Media Studies* 62, no. 3 (2023): 60–85.

Griffis, Noelle. "Teenage Moviemaking on the Lower East Side: The Rivington Street Film Club, 1966–1974." In *Screening Race in American Nontheatrical Cinema*, edited by Alyson Field and Marsha Gordon, 271–89. Durham, NC: Duke University Press, 2019.

Grimaldi, Carmine. "Televising Psyche: Therapy, Play, and the Seduction of Video." *Representations* 139, no. 1 (2017): 95–117.

Halleck, DeeDee. *Hand-Held Visions: The Impossible Possibilities of Community Media*. New York: Fordham University Press, 2002.

Halsell, Grace. *Soul Sister*. New York: Fawcett Crest, 1969.

Hardison, Ayesha. "Theorizing Jane Crow, Theorizing Literary Fragments." *Social Epistemology Review and Reply Collective* 7, no. 2 (2018): 56–73.

Hare, A. Paul, and June Robson Hare. *J. L. Moreno*. London: Sage, 1996.

Harris, LaShawn. *Sex Workers, Psychics, and Number Runners: Black Women in New York City's Underground Economy*. Urbana: University of Illinois Press, 2016.

Hayles, N. Katherine. *How We Became Posthuman: Virtual Bodies in Cybernetics, Literature, and Informatics*. Chicago: University of Chicago Press, 2008.

Hedlund, James. "Computers in Mental Health: An Historical Overview and Summary of Current Status." Second Annual Symposium on Computer Application in Medical Care, 1978 Proceedings (1978), 168–83.

Hicks, Cheryl. *Talk with You Like a Woman: African American Women, Justice, and Reform in New York, 1890–1935*. Chapel Hill: University of North Carolina Press, 2010.

Hill, Reuben, J. Mayone Stycos, and Kurt Back. *The Family and Population Control: A Puerto Rican Experiment in Social Change*. Chapel Hill: University of North Carolina Press, 1959.

Hookway, Branden. "Cockpit." In *Cold War Hothouses*, edited by Beatriz Colomina, Annmarie Brennan, and Jeannie Kim, 22–54. New York: Princeton Architectural Press, 2004.

Hummel, Thomas J., James W. Lichtenberg, and Warren F. Shaffer. "CLIENT 1: A Computer Program Which Simulates Client Behavior in an Initial Interview." *Journal of Counseling Psychology* 22, no. 2 (1975): 164–69.

Inbar, Michael, and Clarice S. Stoll. *Simulation and Gaming in Social Science.* New York: Free Press, 1972.

Jacoby, Irving, and Robert Anderson. "Scenario for Psychiatry." In *Ideas on Film: A Handbook for the 16mm Film User,* edited by Cecile Starr, 42–45. New York: Funk and Wagnalls, 1950.

Jardini, David. "Out of the Blue Yonder: The Transfer of Systems Thinking from the Pentagon to the Great Society, 1961–1965." In *Systems, Experts, and Computers: The Systems Approach in Management and Engineering, World War II and After,* edited by Agatha Hughes and Thomas Hughes, 311–57. Cambridge, MA: MIT Press, 2000.

Jefferson, Brian. *Digitize and Punish: Racial Criminalization in the Digital Age.* Minneapolis: University of Minnesota Press, 2020.

J. G. B. "Coming Through Your Front Door: Prerecorded Video Cassettes." *American Libraries* 1, no. 11 (1970): 1069–73.

Kane, Carolyn L. "The Tragedy of Radical Subjectivity: From Radical Software to Proprietary Subjects." *Leonardo* 47, no. 5 (2014): 480–87.

Kaplan, Seymour R., and Melvin Roman. *The Organization and Delivery of Mental Health Services in the Ghetto: The Lincoln Hospital Experience.* New York: Praeger, 1973.

Kaplan, Wendy, ed. *California Design: 1930–1965: "Living in a Modern Way."* Cambridge, MA: MIT Press, 2011.

Kim, Jina. "Toward a Crip-of-Color Critique: Thinking with Minich's 'Enabling Whom?'" *Lateral* 6, no. 1 (2017).

Knoblauch, Joy. *The Architecture of Good Behavior: Psychology and Modern Institutional Design in Postwar America.* Pittsburgh: University of Pittsburgh Press, 2020.

Korall, Burt. *Drummin' Men: The Heartbeat of Jazz: The Bebop Years.* New York: Oxford University Press, 2002.

Laing, R. D. *The Politics of Experience.* New York: Pantheon Books, 1967.

Lapp, Michael. "The Rise and Fall of Puerto Rico as a Social Laboratory, 1945–1965." *Social Science History* 19, no. 2 (July 1995): 169–99.

Lasch-Quinn, Elisabeth. *Race Experts: How Racial Etiquette, Sensitivity Training, and New Age Therapy Hijacked the Civil Rights Revolution.* New York: W. W. Norton, 2001.

Lea, Andrew M. *Digitizing Diagnosis: Medicine, Minds, and Machines in Twentieth-Century America.* Chapel Hill: University of North Carolina Press, 2023.

LeFrançois, Brenda A., Robert Menzies, and Geoffrey Reaume, eds. *Mad Matters: A Critical Reader in Canadian Mad Studies.* Toronto: Canadian Scholars' Press, 2013.

Lehman, Stanley, Elmer Struening, and M. E. Darling. "Lincoln Hospital Community Mental Health Center: The Development of SARK: An Automated Record-Keeping System for Neighborhood Service Centers." In *Community Mental Health Data Systems: A Description of Existing Programs,* 101–63. Washington, DC: Department of Health, Education, and Welfare, Public Health Service, Health Services, 1970.

Leys, Ruth. *The Ascent of Affect: Genealogy and Critique*. Chicago: University of Chicago Press, 2017.

Lichtenberg, James W., Thomas J. Hummel, and Warren F. Shaffer. "CLIENT 1: A Computer Simulation for Use in Counselor Education and Research." *Counselor Education and Supervision* 24, no. 2 (1984): 155–67.

Light, Jennifer S. *From Warfare to Welfare: Defense Intellectuals and Urban Problems in Cold War America*. Baltimore: Johns Hopkins University Press, 2003.

MacKenzie, Scott. "'Mental Prophylaxis': Crawley Films, McGraw-Hill Educational Films, and Orphan Cinema." In *Cinephemera: Archives, Ephemeral Cinema, and New Screen Histories in Canada*, edited by Zoë Druick and Gerda Cammaer, 59–72. Montreal: McGill-Queen's University Press, 2014.

Markowitz, Gerald, and David Rosner. *Children, Race, and Power: Kenneth and Mamie Clark's Northside Center*. New York: Routledge, 2013.

Massood, Paula. *Black City Cinema: African American Urban Experiences in Film*. Philadelphia, PA: Temple University Press, 2011.

Massood, Paula. *Making a Promised Land: Harlem in Twentieth-Century Photography and Film*. New Brunswick, NJ: Rutgers University Press, 2013.

Materre, Michelle. "Capture and Release: Curating and Exhibiting the East Coast Independent Black Film Movement, 1968–1992." *Black Camera* 10, no. 2 (2019): 149–52.

McIlwain, Charlton D. *Black Software: The Internet and Racial Justice, from the Afro-Net to Black Lives Matter*. New York: Oxford University Press, 2019.

McKinney, Cait. *Information Activism: A Queer History of Lesbian Media Technologies*. Durham, NC: Duke University Press, 2020.

McPherson, Tara. "US Operating Systems at Mid-Century." In *Race After the Internet*, edited by Lisa Nakamura and Peter Chow-White, 21–37. New York: Routledge, 2012.

McRuer, Robert. "In Focus: Cripping Cinema and Media Studies: Introduction." *Journal of Cinema and Media Studies* 58, no. 4 (2019): 134–39.

Menne, Jeff. "Hitchcock's Closed Systems." *Post45*, no. 6 (March 2021). https://post45.org/2021/03/hitchcocks-closed-systems/.

Metzl, Jonathan. *The Protest Psychosis: How Schizophrenia Became a Black Disease*. New York: Beacon Press, 2010.

Mills, Mara. "On Disability and Cybernetics: Helen Keller, Norbert Wiener, and the Hearing Glove." *differences* 22, no. 2–3 (2011): 74–111.

Mitchell, David, and Sharon Snyder. *Narrative Prosthesis: Disability and the Dependencies of Discourse*. Ann Arbor: University of Michigan Press, 2001.

Morales, Iris. *Through the Eyes of Rebel Women: The Young Lords, 1969–1976*. New York: Red Sugarcane Press, 2016.

Moreno, Jacob. *Autobiography of a Genius*. Edited by Edward Schreiber, Sarah Kelley, and Scott Giacomucci. Manchester: North-West Psychodrama Association, 2019.

Moreno, Jacob. "Psychodrama in Action." *Group Psychotherapy* 18, nos. 1–2 (1965): 87–117.

Moreno, Jacob. *Who Shall Survive? A New Approach to the Problem of Human Interrelations*. Washington, DC: Nervous and Mental Disease Publishing Company, 1934.

Moreno, Jacob. *Who Shall Survive? Foundations of Sociometry, Group Psychotherapy and Sociodrama*. New York: Beacon House, 1953.

Morse, Fannie French. "The Farm as a Factor in Training Delinquent Girls." In *Board of Managers, Twenty-First Annual Report of the Board of Managers of the New York State Training School for Girls at Hudson, N.Y., for the Year Ending June 30, 1924*, 20–24. Albany, NY: J. B. Lyon Company, 1924.

Moynihan, Daniel P. *The Negro Family: The Case for National Action*. Washington, DC: Office of Policy Planning and Research, US Department of Labor, 1965.

Mullan, Fitzhugh. *White Coat, Clenched Fist: The Political Education of an American Physician*. Ann Arbor: University of Michigan Press, 2006.

Mumford, Kevin J. "Untangling Pathology: The Moynihan Report and Homosexual Damage, 1965–1975." *Journal of Policy History* 24, no. 1 (2012): 53–73.

Muñoz, José Esteban. *Disidentifications: Queers of Color and the Performance of Politics*. Minneapolis: University of Minnesota Press, 1999.

Muoio, David. "Apple and UCLA Kick Off Device-Driven Depression and Anxiety Study." *mobihealthnews*, August 5, 2020. Last accessed August 31, 2023. https://www.mobihealthnews.com/news/apple-ucla-kick-device-driven-depression-and-anxiety-study.

Murphy, J. J. "The Documentary as Sociodrama: William Greaves's *In the Company of Men* (1969) and *The Deep North* (1988)." In *William Greaves: Filmmaking as Mission*, edited by Scott MacDonald and Jacqueline Najuma Stewart, 197–205. New York: Columbia University Press, 2021.

Murphy, J. J. *Rewriting Indie Cinema: Improvisation, Psychodrama, and the Screenplay*. New York: Columbia University Press, 2019.

Nash, Robert M. "Compliance of Hospitals and Health Agencies with Title VI of the Civil Rights Act." *American Journal of Public Health* 58, no. 2 (1968): 246–51.

Neher, Jack. "Review of *In the Company of Men*." *Psychiatric Services* 22, no. 1 (1971): 31a–32.

Neher, Jack. "Review of *Storefront*." *Psychiatric Services* 19, no. 4 (1968): 125.

Neher, Jack. "Review of *Uptown*." *Psychiatric Services* 17, no. 7 (1966): 218-a.

Nelson, Jennifer. *Women of Color and the Reproductive Rights Movement*. New York: NYU Press, 2003.

New Architecture for Mental Health; New York State Health and Mental Hygiene Improvement Corporation—Report to the Governor. Albany, NY: New York State Health and Mental Hygiene Improvement Corporation, 1969.

Nichols, Bill. "Newsreel: Documentary Filmmaking on the American Left (1971–1975)." PhD diss., University of California, Los Angeles, 1978.

Nicholson, Stuart. *Ella Fitzgerald: A Biography of the First Lady of Jazz*. New York: Da Capo Press, 1995.

Nolte, John. *The Philosophy, Theory and Methods of J. L. Moreno: The Man Who Tried to Become God*. London: Routledge, 2014.

O'Connor, Alice. *Poverty Knowledge: Social Science, Social Policy, and the Poor in Twentieth-Century U.S. History*. Politics and Society in Twentieth-Century America. Princeton, NJ: Princeton University Press, 2001.

Orlando, Norma Jean. "The Mock Ward: A Study in Simulation." In *Behavior Disorders: Perspectives and Trends*, edited by Ohmer Milton and Robert Wahler, 162–70. Philadelphia: Lippincott, 1973.

Orr, Jackie. "Biopsychiatry and the Informatics of Diagnosis: Governing Mentalities." In *Biomedicalization: Technoscience, Health, and Illness in the U.S.*, edited by Adele E. Clarke, Laura Mamo, Jennifer Ruth Fosket, Jennifer R. Fishman, and Janet K. Shim, 353–79. Durham, NC: Duke University Press, 2010.

Orr, Jackie. *Panic Diaries: A Genealogy of Panic Disorder*. Durham, NC: Duke University Press, 2006.

Ostherr, Kirsten. *Medical Visions: Producing the Patient Through Film, Television, and Imaging Technologies*. Oxford: Oxford University Press, 2013.

Ouellette, Laurie. *Viewers Like You: How Public TV Failed the People*. New York: Columbia University Press, 2012.

Parascandola, John. "Syphilis at the Cinema: Medicine and Morals in VD Films of the US Public Health Service in World War II." In *Medicine's Moving Pictures: Medicine, Health, and Bodies in American Film and Television*, edited by Leslie J. Reagan, Nancy Tomes, and Paula A. Treichler, 71–92. Rochester, NY: University of Rochester Press, 2007.

Peavy, Charles. "Pop Art and the Black Revolution: Julian Moreau's The Black Commandos." *Journal of Popular Culture* 3, no. 2 (1969): 205–13.

Peck, Harris, and Elmer Struening. "A Community Mental Health Program in an Urban Slum." In *Mental Health Program Reports*, vol. 2. National Institute of Mental Health, 1968.

Pickens, Therí Alyce. *Black Madness :: Mad Blackness*. Durham, NC: Duke University Press, 2019.

Rankin, Joy Lisi. *A People's History of Computing in the United States*. Cambridge, MA: Harvard University Press, 2018.

Raser, John R. *Simulation and Society: An Exploration of Scientific Gaming*. Boston: Allyn and Bacon, 1969.

Reger, Greg, et al. "Virtual Standardized Patients for Mental Health Education." *Current Psychiatry Reports* 23 (2021): 57–64.

Reichert, Ramon. "Behaviorism, Animation, and Effective Cinema: The McGraw-Hill Industrial Management Film Series and the Visual Culture of Management." In *Films That Work: Industrial Film and the Productivity of Media*, edited by Vinzenz Hediger and Patrick Vondereau, 283–302. Amsterdam: Amsterdam University Press, 2009.

Renov, Michael. "Newsreel: Old and New—Towards an Historical Profile." *Film Quarterly* 41, no. 1 (1987): 20–33.

Reynolds, P. Preston. "The Federal Government's Use of Title VI and Medicare to Racially Integrate Hospitals in the United States, 1963 through 1967." *American Journal of Public Health* 87, no. 11 (1997): 1850–58.

Richert, Lucas. *Break on Through: Radical Psychiatry and the American Counterculture*. Cambridge, MA: MIT Press, 2019.

Robé, Chris. "Detroit Rising: The League of Revolutionary Black Workers, Newsreel, and the Making of *Finally Got the News*." *Film History* 28, no. 4 (2016): 125–58.

Rodriguez-Trías, Helen. "The Hospital as a Community Facility: The Medical Staff and the Hospital." *Bulletin of the New York Academy of Medicine* 48, no. 11 (1972): 1423–27.

Rossi-Snook, Elena, and Lauren Tilton. "'Don't Be a Segregationist: Program Films for Everyone': The New York Public Library's Film Library and Youth Workshops." In *Screening Race in American Nontheatrical Cinema*, edited by Alyson Field and Marsha Gordon, 254–70. Durham, NC: Duke University Press, 2019.

Sager, Clifford, Thomas L. Brayboy, and Barbara R. Waxenberg. *Black Ghetto Family in Therapy: A Laboratory Experience*. New York: Grove Press, 1970.

Sanchez, Sonia. "A Poem for Ella Fitzgerald." In *Like the Singing Coming Off the Drums*, 104–108. New York: Beacon Press, 1998.

Schalk, Sami. "Black Disability Gone Viral: A Critical Race Approach to Inspiration Porn." CLA *Journal* 64, no. 1 (2021): 100–120.

Schalk, Sami. "The Black Disability Politics of the Black Panther Party's Fight Against Psychiatric Abuse." Paper presented at the annual conference of the American Studies Association, November 2019.

Schalk, Sami, and Jina B. Kim. "Integrating Race, Transforming Feminist Disability Studies." *Signs: Journal of Women in Culture and Society* 46, no. 1 (2020): 31–55.

Siegert, Bernard. *Cultural Techniques: Grids, Filters, Doors, and Other Articulations of the Real*. Translated by Geoffrey Winthrop-Young. New York: Fordham University Press, 2014.

Soares, Kristie. "Joy, Rage, and Activism: The Gendered Politics of Affect in the Young Lords Party." *Signs: Journal of Women in Culture and Society* 46, no. 4 (2021): 939–62.

Somerville, Siobhan. *Queering the Color Line: Race and the Invention of Homosexuality in American Culture*. Durham, NC: Duke University Press, 2000.

Spigel, Lynn. TV *by Design: Modern Art and the Rise of Network Television*. Chicago: University of Chicago Press, 2008.

Spigel, Lynn. "Back to the Drawing Board: Graphic Design and the Visual Environment of Television at Midcentury." *Cinema Journal* 55, no. 4 (2016): 28–54.

Spillers, Hortense. "Mama's Baby, Papa's Maybe: An American Grammar Book." *Diacritics* 17, no. 2 (1987): 65–81.

Spitzer, Robert L. "DIAGNO: A Computer Program for Psychiatric Diagnosis Utilizing the Differential Diagnostic Procedure." *Archives of General Psychiatry* 18, no. 6 (1968): 746–56.

Spitzer, Robert L., and Jean Endicott. "DIAGNO II: Further Developments in a Computer Program for Psychiatric Diagnosis." *American Journal of Psychiatry* 125, no. 7S (1969): 12–21.

Sprehe, J. T., and R. L. Michielutte. "Simulation of Social Mobility: Toward the Development of a System of Social Accounts." Paper prepared for the "Theoretical and Methodological Issues" section of the annual meeting of the Eastern Sociological Society, 1969.

Starkweather, J. A., Michael Kamp, and A. Monto. "Psychiatric Interview Simulation by Computer." *Methods of Information in Medicine* 6, no. 1 (1967): 15–23.

Staub, Michael E. *Madness Is Civilization: When the Diagnosis Was Social, 1948–1980*. Chicago: University of Chicago Press, 2011.

Strobel, Charles, Walter Bennett, Peter Ericson, and Bernard Glueck Jr. "Designing

Psychiatric Computer Information Systems: Problems and Strategy." *Comprehensive Psychiatry* 8, no. 6 (1967): 491–508.

Struening, Elmer, Judith Rabkin, and Harris Peck. "Migration and Ethnic Membership in Relation to Social Problems." *American Behavioral Scientist* 13, no. 1 (1969): 57–87.

Summers, Martin. *Madness in the City of Magnificent Intentions: A History of Race and Mental Illness in the Nation's Capital*. New York: Oxford University Press, 2019.

Taylor, Keeanga-Yamahtta. *Race for Profit: How Banks and the Real Estate Industry Undermined Black Homeownership*. Chapel Hill: University of North Carolina Press, 2019.

Underman, Kelly. *Feeling Medicine: How the Pelvic Exam Shapes Medical Training*. New York: NYU Press, 2020.

Visperas, Cristina Mejia. *Skin Theory: Visual Culture and the Postwar Prison Laboratory*. New York: NYU Press, 2022.

Wald, Gayle. *Crossing the Line: Racial Passing in Twentieth-Century US Literature and Culture*. Durham, NC: Duke University Press, 2000.

Walker, Janet. *Couching Resistance: Women, Film, and Psychoanalytic Psychiatry*. Minneapolis: University of Minnesota Press, 1993.

Weinstein, Deborah. *The Pathological Family: Postwar America and the Rise of Family Therapy*. Ithaca, NY: Cornell University Press, 2013.

Weizenbaum, Joseph. "ELIZA—a Computer Program for the Study of Natural Language Communication Between Man and Machine." *Communications of the ACM* 9, no. 1 (1966): 36–45.

Wells, Christi. "'A Dreadful Bit of Silliness': Feminine Frivolity and Ella Fitzgerald's Early Critical Reception." *Women and Music: A Journal of Gender and Culture* 21 (2017): 43–65.

Wells, Christi. "Go Harlem: Chick Webb and His Dancing Audience During the Great Depression." PhD diss., Department of Music, University of North Carolina at Chapel Hill, 2014.

White, Graham, Shane White, Stephen Garton, and Stephen Robertson. *Playing the Numbers: Gambling in Harlem Between the Wars*. Cambridge, MA: Harvard University Press, 2010.

Whooley, Owen. *On the Heels of Ignorance: Psychiatry and the Politics of Not Knowing*. Chicago: University of Chicago Press, 2019.

Williamson, Bess. *Accessible America*. New York: NYU Press, 2019.

Wilmer, Harry A. "Feedback: TV Monologue Psychotherapy." *Radical Software* 1, no. 4 (1971): 11.

Wilmer, Harry A. "Innovative Uses of Videotape on a Psychiatric Ward." *Psychiatric Services* 19, no. 5 (1968): 129–33.

Wilmer, Harry A. "Television: Technical and Artistic Aspects of Videotape in Psychiatric Teaching." *Journal of Nervous and Mental Disease* 144, no. 3 (1967): 207–23.

Wilmer, Harry A. "Television: Technical and Artistic Aspects of Videotape in Psychiatric Teaching." In *Videotape Techniques in Psychiatric Training and Treatment*, edited by Milton Berger, 211–52. New York: Brunner/Mazel, 1970.

Wilmer, Harry A. "Television as Participant Recorder." *American Journal of Psychiatry* 124, no. 9 (1968): 1157–63.

Wilson, Stephen. "Review of GHETTO." *Teaching Sociology* 2, no. 2 (1975): 228–30.

Womack, Autumn. *The Matter of Black Living: The Aesthetic Experiment of Racial Data, 1880–1930*. Chicago: University of Chicago Press, 2022.

Young, Cynthia A. *Soul Power: Culture, Radicalism, and the Making of a US Third World Left*. Durham, NC: Duke University Press, 2006.

Zeavin, Hannah. *The Distance Cure: A History of Teletherapy*. Cambridge, MA: MIT Press, 2021.

Index

www.ingramcontent.com/pod-product-compliance
Lightning Source LLC
Chambersburg PA
CBHW030851270326
41928CB00008B/1318